The Art and Practice
of Low Vision

The Art and Practice of Low Vision

Second Edition

Paul B. Freeman, O.D., F.A.A.O., F.C.O.V.D.
Diplomate in Low Vision

Randall T. Jose, O.D., F.A.A.O.
Diplomate in Low Vision

with special contributions by
Gregory L. Goodrich, Ph.D., F.A.A.O.
Research Diplomate in Low Vision

Jay M. Cohen, O.D., F.A.A.O.
Diplomate in Low Vision

Ian L. Bailey, O.D., M.S., F.A.A.O.
Diplomate in Low Vision

with a foreword by
Eleanor E. Faye, M.D., F.A.C.S.
Consultant, Lighthouse, Inc., New York

Photographs by Katie Jose

Butterworth–Heinemann
Boston   Oxford   Johannesburg   Melbourne   New Delhi   Singapore

Library of Congress Cataloging-in-Publication Data

Freeman, Paul B.
   The art and practice of low vision / Paul B. Freeman, Randall T.
Jose; with special contributions by Greg Goodrich, Jay Cohen, Ian
Bailey; photos by Katie Jose. -- 2nd ed.
      p.   cm.
   Includes bibliographical references and index.
   ISBN 0-7506-9685-0
   1. Low vision--Patients--Rehabilitation. 2. Optometry.   I. Jose,
Randall T., 1943-   . II. Title.
   [DNLM: 1. Vision, Subnormal--diagnosis. 2. Vision, Subnormal-
-rehabilitation.   WW 140F855a 1997]
RE91.F67 1997
617.7--dc21
DNLM/DLC
for Library of Congress   97-12273
                                                                  CIP

British Library Cataloguing-in-Publication Data
A catalogue record for this book is available from the British Library.

The publisher offers special discounts on bulk orders of this book.
For information, please contact:

Manager of Special Sales
Butterworth–Heinemann
313 Washington Street
Newton, MA 02158-1626
Tel: 617-928-2500
Fax: 617-928-2620

For information on all Butterworth–Heinemann publications available,
contact our World Wide Web home page at: http://www.bh.com

10 9 8 7 6 5 4 3 2

Printed in the United States of America

Contents

Contributing Authors

Ian L. Bailey, O.D., M.S., F.A.A.O., Diplomate in Low Vision
Professor of Optometry, University of California, Berkeley

Jay M. Cohen, O.D., F.A.A.O., Diplomate in Low Vision
Professor of Optometry, State University of New York—State College of Optometry, New York

Paul B. Freeman, O.D., F.A.A.O., F.C.O.V.D., Diplomate in Low Vision
Adjunct Faculty, Pennsylvania College of Optometry, Philadelphia; Chief of Low Vision Services, Department of Ophthalmology, Allegheny General Hospital, Pittsburgh

Gregory L. Goodrich, Ph.D., F.A.A.O., Research Diplomate in Low Vision
Research Psychologist, Psychology Service and Western Blind Rehabilitation Center, Palo Alto Health Care System, United States Department of Veterans Affairs, Palo Alto, California; Assistant Clinical Professor of Optometry, University of California, Berkeley

Randall T. Jose, O.D., F.A.A.O., Diplomate in Low Vision
Associate Professor of Vision Rehabilitation, University of Houston College of Optometry; Director of Clinical Services, Houston Delta Gamma Foundation Low Vision Clinic

Foreword

This book is for general practitioners who include low vision patients in their practice, but haven't discovered the secret of being happy doing this work. This book is also for practitioners who may have considered low vision work but have no idea how to start up or organize such a practice.

The emphasis of this book is on organizing an office to cope with the problems and feelings of low vision patients and on incorporating the care of low vision patients into a general practice structure. If we understand the psychological problems of a person with impaired vision, we can create an atmosphere in the office that is reassuring. If we direct the examination, instruction, and prescription toward helping the patient adjust, we are fulfilling the goal of vision rehabilitation.

Whether the practitioner is an "old hand" or a newcomer to low vision treatment, these chapters offer many practical suggestions. I have found the use of model letters, referral sources, community resources, and checklists to be invaluable. Letters are used to introduce patients to low vision procedures, and to help patients develop a much more realistic attitude toward the low vision experience. Other letters can be used to thank people for referrals. When you are very busy, you may neglect to promptly dictate a "thanks-for-the-referral" letter. With an attractive model letter, the details can be filled in quickly, and the thank-you letter can be on the way in the next mail.

This book does not try to do any more than outline the ingredients of the examination, the essential function tests, and the equipment and devices needed. Techniques are suggested, but the choice is left to the individual practitioner and style of practice.

The wide selection of home training sheets are invaluable for treating patients who need this type of reinforcement.

The emphasis of this book is on the patient, as it should be. By filling out pre-examination and history forms, the patient develops a reality base that saves the practitioner a lot of unnecessary backtracking to undo unrealistic expectations. While reviewing this material, I was reminded of how easy it is to forget how lost and frustrated a new patient feels and how long it takes to adjust. The average clinician cannot and should not spend lengthy sessions with a patient. Nor can an instructor be expected to pick up clues immediately. But if the patient has time to review and think over the material provided in advance, the therapeutic process can take place where it should—in the patient's own mind, with support from those persons close to the patient. Working with family or friends introduces another type of reinforcement for the patient—that of a family relationship or a shared activity with a friend.

Rehabilitation does not always lead to happy patients, but the well-informed person who participates fully in his or her therapy learns to accept and work with his or her limitations with a better understanding.

The Art and Practice of Low Vision is what its title says it is. It does not attempt to introduce yet another method of treating low vision, but rather tries to fill in the important spaces that are generally glossed over in texts on low vision—that is, how to make the treatment of low vision fit into a busy practice and be successful and satisfying.

Eleanor E. Faye, M.D., F.A.C.S.

Preface to the First Edition

The Art and Practice of Low Vision is a how-to book for the clinician who wants either to begin or enhance a low vision practice.

This book walks the practitioner through the steps of a low vision practice. We provide forms and handouts that should not only make the clinician's venture into a low vision practice easier, but also provide optimum care for patients. The concepts presented are based on our clinical experience. For those who wish to understand the more academic aspects of the clinical information presented, we direct your attention to Appendix D, which lists additional bibliographic resources and materials.

The primary goal of a low vision patient who seeks help is usually to be able to read again. The ability to read print is an important part of an individual's effort to maintain an independent life. However, many low vision patients misunderstand the nature of the help they can get from optical devices and quickly become discouraged. They often confuse the ability to recognize letters with the ability to read.

It is a thrilling moment when a person who is visually impaired sits in an examination chair, looks through a pair of lenses, and actually sees letters again. But, of course, reading requires much more—speed, fluency, comprehension—and it may take months of practice to attain these skills. Recognition of individual reading goals is also required; they may differ from person to person. One patient may want to be able to read the directions for knitting a sweater without having to ask for help, while another may want to read several mystery novels a week. Their vision may be identical, but it may take considerably more effort on the part of the latter patient to achieve the desired goal.

Although the primary goal of a low vision patient is often reading, many also want to view objects in the distance (e.g., bus signs, television, fast-food wall menus, or friends' faces). It is exciting for a visually impaired person to see 20/20, but seeing a stationary chart and becoming visually functional are worlds apart.

The goal of the low vision practitioner is to help low vision patients understand the nature of the rehabilitative process and to help them meet their individual goals whenever possible. This is achieved by providing careful evaluations of the impairment, making relevant recommendations for low vision devices, suggesting exercises that will assist patient progress, and tracking this progress through follow-up examinations.

We hope this book will serve as a starting point for many low vision or potential low vision practitioners. With increased experience and patient contact, the information from this book will further enhance patient care.

PBF
RTJ

Preface to the Second Edition

Before undertaking any task in optometry one should have a philosophy of care. The philosophy of care or mission statement should reflect you and your practice. After years of not realizing this, I had the opportunity to spend time at a hotel with a national presence. The staff there was unlike any hotel staff I had ever encountered. After being treated like royalty (as was everyone else) and having staff members refuse tips for doing what they considered their job, I inquired as to how all of this could be true. The manager gave me a copy of their mission statement.

This experience prompted me to think about what my own mission statement might be. The mission statement on the following page is what developed. Please use this, modify it, or develop your own. The meaning of these statements is what the reader decides.

PBF

MISSION STATEMENT

- *We are eye care professionals helping those who are visually impaired to choose visual options to obtain a goal and maintain dignity.*

- *We recognize that this evaluation and management is part of the continuum of primary eye care.*

- *We bring to the evaluation honesty, compassion, empathy, and certainty of direction.*

- *We do not prejudge the motivational needs and desires of our patients.*

Acknowledgments

This book could not have been written without the help, either directly or indirectly, of several people. The help of professionals we have worked with during our respective careers in optometry has been invaluable. In the field of low vision, any truly great work is done through a multidisciplinary team effort. The individuals we have worked with exemplify that concept.

We would also like to thank all those who have written in the field of low vision. Without those erudite individuals, works like this could not have been envisioned. We would especially like to thank, as a group, the low vision diplomates of the American Academy of Optometry. It is through interacting with this merry band of concerned practitioners that we were able to bounce many of our ideas around.

This type of work cannot be done without the labor of readers, typists, and all-around helpers. Thanks to Pat Miller for the hours spent helping to do the tough job of reading, rereading, and typing.

Finally, we thank our wives, Barbara and Maryann, who have continued to support us in our academic efforts and helped us keep our sanity through it all.

PBF
RTJ

Introduction

Have you ever wondered where patients go when they have been told nothing more can be done? We hope that by the time you finish reading this book you will not have to answer that question for your patients. Furthermore, you will be able to answer that question for hundreds of patients whose practitioners do not have the opportunity to enhance the quality of life for those with visual impairments that cannot be resolved by conventional medical or optical treatment.

This issue becomes increasingly important as the population ages and average lifespan increases, as medical science saves many of the impaired infants who, in years past, would have succumbed to their disabling diseases, and as more people of all ages become survivors of traumatic brain injury and closed-head trauma that may create multiple disabilities. All of these groups have potential for visual impairments that cannot be helped conventionally but can be helped by the low vision clinician.

Before examining a low vision patient, you should be familiar with certain terminology, equipment, and managerial information.

Definition of Services

You must be able to define what a low vision examination is and what a low vision examination is not. Following is a definition to consider when explaining to your patients, their families, third-party payors, and others what you do, why it is different from a primary examination, and why a team approach may be necessary.

What a Low Vision Examination Is

A low vision examination is an optical and functional evaluation to determine whether the patient's vision can be enhanced to enable the patient to participate in desired activities. The examination should include an exploration of optical and nonoptical systems, in addition to the patient's perceptual and physiologic skills. When coordinated with other optometric, medical, educational, and rehabilitative services, the end results should enable the patient to maximize his or her sight.

To set the stage for that process, a low vision refraction must be performed when conventional refractive techniques have been tried and failed. The use of radical retinoscopic techniques, subjective testing with trial frame, trial lenses, telescopes, and other distance optical devices; modified optotypes; target positioning; lighting; and other visual modifiers are used to determine the following:

1. Whether a conventional lens can be appropriately modified, not necessarily for quantitative measurements, but for improved qualitative acuities.

2. Whether a conventional lens prescription, in combination with additional distance optics (e.g., telescopes, electro-optical systems), near optics (e.g., microscopes, hand-held and stand magnifiers, electro-optical systems), field-awareness systems (e.g., mirrors, prisms, reversed telescopes), or nonoptical devices could be used to improve sight and visual performance.

What a Low Vision Examination Is Not

A low vision examination is not a medical evaluation to determine eye health. Such an evaluation should be performed by the referring practitioner as justification for additional specialized services. It is imperative that the patient have a primary care optometrist or ophthalmologist who can monitor any eye conditions that could result in eye health problems or further vision loss. Patients should always be encouraged to return to the primary care eye doctor for continued care at regular intervals.

A medical evaluation, however, may often be performed in conjunction with a low vision evaluation. Any existing disease should be monitored for change so that appropriate medical care can be provided as quickly as possible. Delaying care can mean the difference between being able to minimize disease-related sight changes and losing remaining vision to disease. Obviously, the latter case would also negatively impact the rehabilitation program. There are also situations in which surgical intervention is appropriate to facilitate the rehabilitation process (e.g., cataract surgery). If a patient enters the low vision practice office as a primary care patient, all appropriate diagnostic and therapeutic activities (within the scope of the practitioner's license) should be performed before the low vision assessment begins.

Scheduling

Scheduling a low vision patient can be tricky because the patient's first visit must incorporate a number of concerns: the patient's expectations, basic findings, a summary of what has been done, the direction the patient wishes to pursue, and so forth. Typically, initial evaluations should be allotted 1.0–1.5 hours. If the evaluation is finished earlier than scheduled, the remaining time can be used to discuss patient concerns regarding the condition that led to decreased vision, information about practitioner referral, family interaction, and so forth.

Subsequent Scheduling

Subsequent appointments should be scheduled so that additional tests or verification procedures can be completed and low vision therapy or stimulation activities can be provided. These sessions should last 30–45 minutes. Remember that during each visit the patient may provide information that will require modification in the management plan and ultimate prescription. Allow time for these modifications.

Additionally, from both a legal and measurement (monitoring) perspective, some tests need to be performed at every visit. These may include visual acuities, intraocular pressures, and any other tests necessary to monitor the patient's eye health.

Below is a chart that summarizes the movement of low vision patients from initial evaluation to continued care. It may be helpful to make a copy of the chart and post it in your office to remind you and your staff of the proper sequence.

Schedule the patient
History with goal emphasis
Evaluation and management of patient
Summary/goal review/follow-up visit(s)
Telephone call monitoring between visits
Completion of services
Telephone follow-up/monitoring
    At 1 month
    At 3 months
Clinical re-evaluation at 6 months or as needed

Equipment Needs

The primary goal of most patients is to be able to read or perform other near activities. Therefore, near optical systems should be available. Television viewing, shopping, and other distance activities also require evaluation and readily accessible devices. Therefore, telescopes and electro-optical systems for distance should also be available. The following is a list of suggested low vision devices for the typical low vision practitioner. Before building a large stock of systems, however, you should be proficient in prescribing low vision devices. The initial outlay can be as much or as little as you wish.

Equipment

Several companies offer kits for the practitioner starting a low vision practice (e.g., Designs for Vision; Freeman Low Vision Kit; Spalding Magnifiers Inc.; Lighthouse, Inc.; Eschenbach; Mattingly-Jose Kit) Most of the kits incorporate the company's own products. You will eventually need diagnostic equipment in each of the following treatment option areas:

1. Full-field microscopes, +8.00–50.00 D
2. Prismatic half-eyes, +4.00–12.00 D
3. Hand-held magnifiers, +8.00–20.00 D
4. Pocket magnifiers, +16.00–40.00 D
5. Stand magnifiers, +12.00–32.00 D
6. Illuminated stand magnifiers, +24.00–48.00 D
7. Halogen (Xenon) illuminated magnifiers, +24.00–48.00 D
8. Hand-held telescopes, 2.5–10.0×
9. Binocular spectacle telescopes, 3× (galilean focusable)
10. Near binocular telemicroscopes, 2.5–4.0×
11. Bioptics, 2–6× (keplerian focusable)
12. Binoculars (monoculars), 7–18×
13. Filters (NOIR, Corning, etc.)
14. Closed-circuit television (CCTV), Magni-Cam, Low Vision Imaging System (LVIS), V-max
15. Special diagnostic charts
16. Loan system

These kits range in price from a modest $1,000 to meet the occasional primary care need to $20,000 for a comprehensive set to meet all needs (including loaned systems). One of the authors (PBF) has designed the Freeman Low Vision Trial Kit (Designs for Vision) with optical components that are functional but not redundant.

Freeman Low Vision Trial Kit

The Freeman Low Vision Trial Kit includes the following:

Trial glasses assembly—May frame
Trial glasses assembly—Yeoman frame
2.2× Full-diameter telescope, clear (in trial ring)
3.0×, 4.0× Galilean spiral telescopes with adapter
2.0×, 3.0×, 4.0×, 5.0×, and 6.0× Expanded-field telescopes, spiral focusable with adapters
2×, 3×, 4×, 5×, 6×, 7×, and 8× ClearImage II trial rings
8×, 10×, 12×, and 14× ClearImage II 28-mm telephotos
Trial ring assembly
Trial ring assembly—telephoto
Auxiliary holder assemblies—left and right

Occluder cap—adjustable
Hand-held magnifier with adapter
General Electric light meter
Interpupillary distance millimeter ruler
Tape measure assembly
Fitted Samsonite case
Two interpupillary distance centering caps—clear
Two Jackson cross cylinders

Some highlights of the kit are as follows:

1. The telescopes can be used as hand-held telescopes and trial frame telescopes (by using a ring adapter) or in the kit frame, designed to demonstrate how the system looks and is used as a spectacle.

2. The ClearImage lenses can be used in a trial lens frame and in a kit frame for demonstration purposes. This will allow you to evaluate magnification in the +8.00–32.00 D range. The ClearImage lenses can also be used as hand-held magnifiers, by using the hand-held magnifier housing with the well that will accept the Clear-Image lenses (included in the kit).

3. The telephoto lenses can also be used in both the trial lens frame and in the kit frame to demonstrate the use of the system in a more natural manner.

4. The light meter and ruler are included for situations in which illumination and distance measurements are needed. This kit is especially good for those clinicians who will use this system for traveling to other sites outside the primary office.

The Freeman Low Vision Trial Kit is a prepackaged system that allows the low vision practitioner to evaluate most patients and demonstrate magnification that over 90% of the low vision population will appreciate (Figure 1).

Loan System

A loan system is a must. Patients who perform well in the office with a specific device may not perform as well at home. Regardless of how much training is provided in the office, there are environmental considerations the doctor cannot be aware of unless patients take the devices home. Some systems—for example, some electro-optical systems (e.g., CCTV, LVIS, Magni-Cam, V-max) and some of the more sophisticated autofocus telescopes—cannot be easily loaned to the patient. These devices are usually evaluated over numerous, extensive office visits.

The loan system essentially takes away the burden of "forced success." As long as the device is loaned, neither member of the

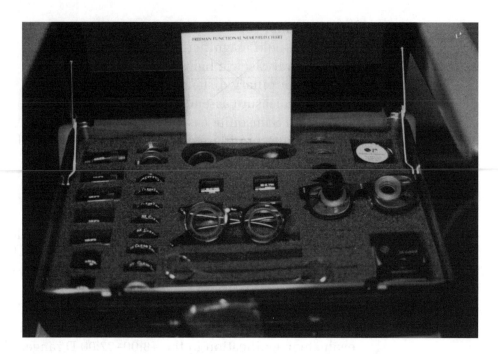

Figure 1. The Designs for Vision Freeman Low Vision Trial Kit provides the optical devices needed to provide excellent low vision care in the office or for off-site programs. It will enable you to demonstrate magnification from 2× to 14× in microscopic, magnifier, and telescopic designs. It is the easiest way to start a low vision practice.

doctor-patient team will feel the pressure to create perceived success. After using a loaned device, a patient can be prescribed a system with first-hand knowledge of its advantages and limitations. If the patient is prescribed a device without a trial period, the doctor might feel the need to continue to "push" the device to avoid giving the patient a refund. Or the patient may feel the doctor has simply sold the device without a proper trial.

The length of time and the fee involved with a loan system depend on you and the patient. There should be (and usually is) a specified time period with any low vision device after which there is a point of diminishing return. This length of time is personalized based on the patient's additional challenges.

Incidentally, the loan system is not unique to low vision practitioners. Many contact lens practitioners use the trial system to determine if a patient will be successful with a particular lens.

You have a number of fiscal options in the loan process depending on the philosophy of your office:

1. Loan the devices at no cost without having the patient sign any form about responsibility of loss, breakage, or extended use.

2. Require patients to pay for the device and return the patient's money if use of the device is not successful after a specified period of time.

3. Loan a device with an agreement for remuneration should the device not be returned on time or not returned at all (Form 1).

4. Charge a user's fee, which may or may not be put toward the cost of the device. By paying this fee, the patient has made a financial commitment to you for at least some coverage should the device be lost. The authors have found that this concept has met with minimal or no resistance. It is also explained that the fee allows the practitioner to exchange systems within a family of devices (e.g., microscopes as a family, telescopes as a family) during training without any additional charge.

The authors have found that options 3 and 4 work best. Neither puts an undue financial burden on a patient who may not experience success with a system. These options give the practitioner the latitude to charge the patient for overdue loaned devices using option 3 or to cover some expenses using option 4.

When a device is prescribed and ordered for a patient the payment policy must again be explained. Extended payment plans are sometimes necessary. Most practitioners have their own system of determining those qualifications.

In some situations loaned devices are not returned regardless of what you do. Typically there are three reasons devices are returned or payments are not completed:

- Death
- The patient does not want to return the device
- The patient feels it is unnecessary to pay

As strange as it may seem, it is not always the unhappy patient or family who chooses not to make a payment. You should have procedures in place to deal with the above situations. We have found the following method to work well:

1. Contact the patient, family, or estate by telephone to request the device or payment.
2. Send a three-option follow-up letter if the telephone call does not produce results (Form 2).
3. Send a final follow-up letter with a message, a warning, and the name of a collection agency (Form 3).
4. Turn the account over to a collection agency.

This system can be structured as tightly or loosely as your practice policies dictate.

Low Vision Staff

Initially a low vision practitioner should conduct every activity required in the low vision evaluation, from intake to evaluation to training. Once the practitioner is comfortable with the total process, other staff members can perform various segments of the evaluation. Using nonophthalmic professional staff (e.g., orientation and mobility instructors, social workers, occupational therapists, physical therapists) is wonderful but not always practical because of scheduling and financial considerations. These services should be available to both you and your patients in the community. When provided in conjunction with the use of low vision devices, however, the additional professional services should be guided by the low vision optometrist or physician.

Fee Structure

Fees can be divided into evaluation, management, and device fees. Evaluation and management billing can be given to the patient before or at the conclusion of the initial evaluation. Fees are frequently broken down for the patient according to services that are covered by insurance and those that are not. You should be familiar with insurance carriers and third-party payors in your area (or where the patient is from) to determine what is covered and what is not. The noncovered portion of the fees should be collected as soon as possible and definitely before any additional activities or loaner devices are given to the patient. Most devices that are prescribed are not typically covered by third-party payors. As a result, the fee for the devices will be the responsibility of the patient. If the patient is unwilling or unable to pay for the portion of the noncovered evaluation, you will have a much better idea about his or her responsibility or capability to pay for other noncovered expenses.

Deciding how to charge and the process for submitting fees to third-party payors is a difficult issue. The fee structure in low vision care should be similar to that of any other aspect of an eye care practice. Before determining a fee, all that goes into an examination should be carefully considered. Look at the policies of government agencies, specifically Medicare, to help determine the complexity of care you offer. Keep in mind that what is covered and what is not should not influence your decision about the degree of complexity of covered services. Meeting with third-party payors to discuss the evaluation will provide guidelines for thinking about your services. Anyone you speak to, however, will interpret the information based on personal knowledge. Review how you might justify your services should you need to do so. Use guidelines given to you by the carriers (e.g., history, examination and medical decision making) when formulating your thoughts.

The patient should be thoroughly informed regarding fees. The explanation of fees can take place at the time of initial phone contact with the patient or family or at the conclusion of the evaluation. When considering discussion of fees before the evaluation, remember that some patients have been told that nothing can be done to improve their vision. Should the prospective patient be surprised by the fee and know that some of it may not be covered by insurance, a visit may not be scheduled. The prospective patient may feel that this evaluation may also lead to a dead end. Then, if the patient's expectations are not met after the evaluation, you will have an unhappy and angry patient. When fees are discussed at the conclusion of the evaluation, after a demonstration of visual success that no one else could provide, however, the patient is usually more receptive to the fee, regardless of who is fiscally responsible. This response also demonstrates that, at least, the patient's expectations have been met.

The decision of fiscal responsibility is based on the questions you are asking. When providing consultation or evaluation to the visually impaired patient, two specific questions must always be asked initially and sometimes as continued visual enhancement care is performed.

The practitioner should first answer this question: *Are there any other forms of medical treatment that could help the patient?* The response is more sophisticated and challenging when asked about a low vision patient as opposed to a visually healthy patient. Low vision patients will not return to normal or near normal acuities or visual fields even with medical intervention. They have been previously evaluated and determined to have no standard medical-surgical therapy options and are referred to you to address the medical problem through low vision intervention and devices. Typically, everything else has been tried. The buck stops with you. Some examples may be helpful in understanding the complexity of this question:

1. Patient 1 has 20/400 vision due to macular degeneration and cataracts. He just visited a practitioner who told him the cataracts should not be removed because his vision will not be improved by this procedure. He has been referred to a low vision practitioner to determine whether low vision devices will help.

The low vision practitioner must answer this question: If the cataracts are removed before a low vision evaluation is performed or during the course of low vision care, will the visual acuities be enhanced from 20/400 to 20/200 or from a blurry to a clear 20/400?

In a general practice, this thinking may be somewhat foreign. However, for the low vision practitioner, this information may lead to the modification of the design of the low vision device and recommendations for lighting, contrast, and other potential nonoptical enhancement conditions. The medical decision making should be reviewed by the low vision practitioner and patient. Suggestions can then be made to the referring doctor, or the patient can be referred to a primary care doctor who can carry out the procedure if warranted. The practitioner asked to perform the surgery should be informed that the patient is not expecting a miracle and that the surgery is going to produce a clearer (rather than hazy) blur, allowing for a more successful enhancement of remaining vision through low vision services.

In some instances, the primary care doctor may suggest that surgery not be attempted until all optical and nonoptical options have been pursued and found completely unacceptable. This may be the case for a patient who had cataract surgery in one eye and the result was only light perception. In this situation, the surgeon may want to be conservative about a surgical approach to the other functional eye and use surgery as a last resort. This may also be a medically complex patient, and given the choice, the surgeon would rather avoid surgery that could result in ophthalmic complications or risks to general health.

2.   Patient 2 has diabetic retinopathy and has been referred to a low vision practitioner. Because of diabetic complications, an appointment scheduled for a week after the initial primary care evaluation has been rescheduled for 6 weeks later. The low vision practitioner should evaluate not only the functional goal-oriented information but determine ocular health to confirm that changes have not taken place. Because access to the previous doctor's internal evaluation regarding hemorrhages or apparent reasons for a medical re-evaluation is not always available, any disease observations should be communicated by letter or telephone to the primary care doctor or referred to a primary care doctor based on diabetic guidelines distributed by the American Optometric Association (AOA) and the American Academy of Ophthalmology (AAO). This communication is extremely important not only to provide the best low vision evaluation but also to prevent further loss of vision.

3.   Patient 3 has been diagnosed with macular degeneration and referred to you. On low vision evaluation, she shows an increase in intraocular pressures. This compounds the retinal problem with potential glaucomatous involvement. The low vision practitioner must decide whether to refer her back to the primary care referral source for appropriate treatment or, where appropriate (as in the nonreferred primary care patient), begin treatment as indicated.

To determine which patients have medical complications that can affect visual processing, the low vision practitioner must remember to answer this important question: Are there any other modes of medical treatment that could benefit the patient visually even after the patient has been told nothing more can be done? Keep in mind that this is a more sophisticated version of the same question asked of a general practitioner.

These are only a few examples of potential medical complications that can modify the response to the second question: *Are there any optical or nonoptical options that will help this patient regain lost visual acuities?* This question is addressed by the low vision evaluation.

Third-party payor guidelines typically suggest that tests performed to answer the first question are covered as a medically related decision-making process whereas tests related to the second are typically noncovered and are the patient's fiscal responsibility. However, the practitioner should consult with the patient's carrier to determine which of these services are paid for by insurance.

Patients should also be apprised of third-party reimbursement. Because optometrists have entered into the third-party reimbursement arena, they must understand that third-party carriers follow certain guidelines regardless of the specialty of the doctor. Following are some guidelines to help the optometrist through the third-party payor maze.

1. Third-party payors do not typically cover services included in routine evaluations. Coverage is designed to assist those in need of care due to a medically necessary condition. The low vision patient is a patient with a decreased visual acuity or reduced visual field due to a medically diagnosed condition of the visual system and should fit into most profiles required by third-party payors. It is incumbent upon you, however, to understand the language used by third-party payors before reimbursement to either you or the patient.

2. Low vision services, in almost all instances, are noncovered services. One reason is that there is no coded service with this title. Low vision is not a disease; it is the functional result of a disease. Reimbursement is driven by diagnosis.

3. Most carriers need one diagnosis to reimburse a patient or doctor for the service. Listing more than one diagnosis will not impress the person who enters the information into the computer. In fact, multiple diagnoses could lead to certain tests not being covered, based on confusion about a specific pathology as it relates to services rendered. However, it is probably wise to inquire whether additional diagnostic listings are appropriate. Please note that it is becoming more important to be very specific in your diagnosis and the numerical coding that defines the disease. Many carriers do not accept inappropriate numerical or abbreviated coding.

4. When you are planning to submit a claim for a specific service, first determine whether that service is covered in your locality or where your patient's carrier is based. This can be determined by directly contacting the carrier, the AOA, or the AAO. The AOA and the AAO have diagnostic codes as well as office visit and consultation codes available. Consultative visits, office visits, and the level of those visits are not necessarily covered by all carriers in all sections of the country. Rather than frustrating and embarrassing both you and your patient, it is advisable to clarify which services are covered.

5. For services that are consultative in nature, it is important to review item 4. In addition, a consultation typically applies to the first visit. Any visit following a consultation, according to most carriers, is usually considered an office visit, the complexity of which depends upon the type of service being rendered. To qualify as a consultation, a visit must meet certain requirements, including the following:

- The practitioner renders advice to the patient.
- The practitioner writes a report to the referring doctor. This information must be taken under advisement by the referring doctor in establishing a treatment program.
- The practitioner may, in certain circumstances, begin prescribing at a consultation visit. (If there is a high probability that the practitioner will assume the care of the patient it is generally not considered a consultation. However, always check with the patient's carrier for regional interpretations.)

6. Any special services that you wish to perform and want covered by third-party payors must be justified not only in your mind but also in the mind of the payor. For example, taking a picture of the fundus of a cataract patient when cataract is the diagnosis being used, may not be covered because of the apparent lack of relationship between a fundus photograph and the diagnosis of cataract in the mind of the third-party payor. In the final analysis, anything can be rejected by the third-party payor and then must be justified by you.

7. Using codes in third-party billing that are not optometric/ophthalmic, even if they result in reimbursement, can lead to trouble. Third-party carriers can decide later that they have made a mistake and can come back to you to collect those funds (and possibly interest), even if they were in error. This process is called the *post-payment review.*

8. Using maximum reimbursable codes over multiple visits may send up a red flag, cause the payor to deny payment, or invite a visit from a third-party payor for an explanation of services. An

example of this is the overuse of complex or high-level office visits or consultations. It is assumed that you have provided every available service for each of those visits.

9. Low vision devices are not typically reimbursable. However, some practitioners have tried and been successful in receiving reimbursement by writing a narrative with a diagnosis. However, do not be surprised if the claim is denied.

10. Managed care is a system of reimbursement becoming omnipresent in the provision of health care. Each managed care plan is unique. To obtain maximum benefits for your patients you must learn what each of these plans covers and the steps involved in obtaining authorization for your services and prescribed devices (where applicable). Many of these plans require participation on a panel or coordination of services with a panel member.

These guidelines will be useful in helping you legitimately justify and maximize the use of third-party payors for your benefit and the benefit of your patient. Keep in mind these are only guidelines. The final decision rests with you.

Form 1 (on letterhead)

Patient Receipt and Acknowledgment of Agreement
for Use of Low Vision Device(s)

Patient's name: _____

Date: _____

Low vision device(s): _____

Return date: _____

Daily rental after return date: $ _____

Value of device: $ _____

I have this day received from _____, O.D., the low vision device(s) ("the device") described above. I agree that the device is solely for the use of the above-named patient. I also agree that I will return the device on or before the return date. This return date can only be changed by approval of _____, O.D., in writing. If I do not return the device by the return date, I agree to pay _____, O.D., daily rental in the amount listed above until the device is returned. I also agree to pay _____, O.D., for any damage sustained to the device while it is in my possession.

Witness the execution of this agreement intending to be legally bound.

_____
Date

_____
Patient's name (print name)

_____
(Signature)

Extension Date Approval (please date and initial)

Date			
Patient			
Doctor			

Date: _____

Dear _____:

Our laboratory has brought to our attention that you still have a low vision device out on loan. It has been at least 2 months since we have heard from you. Please respond by doing one of the following:

1. Call the office to make an appointment, or
2. Return the borrowed system(s), or
3. Send a check for the cost of the system: $_____

We would appreciate it if you would take care of this matter as soon as possible. Thank you.

Accounting Department

Form 3

Date: _____
Dear _____ :

Once again, we would like to inform you that your account with this office has been unpaid for several months. We have sent monthly reminders and have made several other attempts to contact you about this unpaid balance.

We always have the well-being of our patients in mind, but at this point we must be fair to ourselves and our other patients. We cannot continue to provide the quality of staff and services that our patients require if we are not paid for them.

Because of the cost of covering an overdue bill and in fairness to patients who have paid their bills, we have no alternative but to refer your account for collection, a step we sincerely regret. Won't you please respond to this last appeal and thus avoid a procedure that can only add to your inconvenience and expense?

We sincerely hope you will respond to this letter. Your account will be turned over to _____ for collection if we do not hear from you within 10 days.

Sincerely,

The Art and Practice
of Low Vision

1 | Before the Initial Examination

The phone rings and a low vision patient or patient's family member makes an appointment or a referring doctor's office schedules a low vision patient for your services. After the appointment has been made, communication is an integral part of your initial contact with the patient. Before the initial examination, you should write several pieces of correspondence.

In this chapter, we examine the kinds of letters you will write. On the following pages are examples of letters and forms you can use to communicate with your patient; the referring doctor or source; and the patient's spouse, family member, or helper. You can also design your own correspondence using these as guides.

CONTENTS

1.1 Introductory Letters
1.2 Thank You for the Referral
1.3 Thank You for Your Help
1.4 Brief History
1.5 About Your Appointment

FORM DESCRIPTIONS

1.1 Introductory Letters
The first two letters acquaint patients, referring or blindness agencies, doctors, and others with your facility and process.
  1.1a Form 1.1a is a cover letter for any potential referral source. A pamphlet about the services available at your office should be enclosed.
  1.1b Form 1.1b describes your services to a potential patient.

1.2 Thank You for the Referral
These two letters indicate whether the referred patient has made an appointment.

1.2a   The first letter you need to write is to the referral source. Not only is this good public relations but it also lets the referral source know that the patient has made an appointment.

1.2b   Form 1.2b is extremely important. It notifies the referral source that the referred patient did not keep the appointment. Without this notice, the referral source may feel left out of the loop or believe that the patient has been "lost" to your practice.

1.3   Thank You for Your Help

At the time the appointment is made, determine whether there is a person who can help the prospective patient read the materials you will send before the initial examination. Form 1.3 should accompany the appointment form so the patient's spouse, family member, or helper can help read the information.

1.4   Brief History

With the thank-you letter, enclose a brief history form for the patient to complete.

The point of the brief history is to obtain introductory background information necessary to help you better understand the patient and decide before the appointment what procedural modifications may be necessary to achieve your patient's goals. Many clinicians have a higher vision rehabilitation success rate with patients who complete the brief history form before the initial evaluation. Remember that a more formal history will be taken at the office during the first visit.

1.5   About Your Appointment

Along with the letter and Form 1.4, you should enclose the information contained in Form 1.5. This handout includes instructions about what the patient should bring to the initial examination and provides information about setting realistic treatment goals. Sending these materials in large-print format (i.e., 1.2–2.0 M typeface) may help patients respond independently to the questions, assuring them even before the evaluation that you have thought about potential methods of visual assistance. This is a great boon to good doctor-patient rapport.

Finally, you may want to include a map, public transportation access with phone numbers, and any other information that may make the patient feel more at ease.

Introductory Letter for Potential Referral Source

Dear _____:

At the suggestion of some of the agencies we work with, we are writing to acquaint you with the services available through our office for the care of low vision patients. We have found that through coordinated information and cooperative efforts, many low vision individuals can become more productive and independent.

Enclosed you will find information about our office. Please feel free to stop by and visit us. I am sure you will find your visit both informative and enjoyable. If we can be of further assistance, please do not hesitate to call.

Sincerely,

Enclosure: office pamphlet

Form 1.1b (on letterhead)

Introductory Letter for Potential Patient

Dear _____:

Thank you for inquiring about our low vision services. Your in-office evaluation will include a comprehensive history, a discussion of your specific needs and goals, a review of the cause of your visual impairment, and a complete low vision examination. At the conclusion of the visit, we will review our findings with you and those who have accompanied you. The fee for this visit will be $ _____ . Some insurance policies will defray part of the cost. Please feel free to inquire about this.

Once it has been determined that a low vision device(s) will be useful, a home program to help you learn to use the device(s) may be instituted. You will be monitored for success both at home and in our office. Only after success has been achieved will the device(s) be prescribed.

Care and maintenance instructions will be dispensed with the device(s). Our staff will make periodic phone calls during the first year to assure you that we are available if you need additional guidance in the use or care of your device(s).

Patients generally come to us by referral. It is our policy to send a report to the referral source describing examination results and the type of low vision device(s) that has been prescribed. This information will be important, as we expect all patients to continue to receive care from their family eye doctor.

Many of our patients travel from long distances. We will be glad to arrange overnight accommodations. Because our office is on one of the city's main thoroughfares, public transportation and taxi services are readily available.

If we can be of assistance, please contact us at _____ (phone number).

Sincerely,

4

Thank You for the Referral

Dear _____:

    Thank you for referring _____ for a low vision evaluation._____ is scheduled to be seen on _____.
I will keep you informed of our services as they are provided. Again, thank you for referring _____ and allowing me the opportunity to share in your patient's vision care.

    Sincerely,

Thank You for the Referral

Dear _____:

    Thank you for referring _____ for a consultation and low vision evaluation. _____ was scheduled for an evaluation on _____ . We want to let you know that your patient did not keep this appointment. However, my office will contact your patient to set up another appointment.

    Should we be unable to schedule another appointment, we will contact you again. We will always be happy to see your patient in the future if a referral examination is still desired.

    Sincerely,

Thank You for Your Help

Dear _____:

    This information has been sent to help _____ prepare for a low vision evaluation. Reading this letter may be difficult, if not impossible, for (him/her). I would, and I'm sure _____ would, appreciate your help in reading this. As you read this, you will begin to understand the potential help available for _____ and the procedures that will be involved.

    Thank you in advance for your help.

    Sincerely,

Brief History

Please circle Yes or No for each question.

Can you read print?	Yes	No
Do you use magnifiers?	Yes	No
Can you watch television?	Yes	No
Do you still drive?	Yes	No
Can you travel independently?	Yes	No
Are you taking medications?	Yes	No

If yes, please list.

_____

_____

_____

Does sunlight bother your eyes?	Yes	No
Do you wear sunglasses?	Yes	No

What bothers you the most about your vision loss?

_____

_____

_____

About Your Appointment

WELCOME

You have made an appointment for a low vision examination. This is one of the most important actions you can take to improve your ability to see. This letter will familiarize you with ways you can assist me and my staff as we help you.

First, you must realize there are no miracles. Your lost vision cannot be restored. Low vision care is a rehabilitation process: You are going to be taught to effectively use your remaining vision.

You can be helped to use your remaining vision in three ways.

1. By learning to use your remaining vision more efficiently than you do now. There are some eye movement skills you will learn to help you do this.

2. By using alternative methods to perform certain tasks. These include better lighting; high-contrast, enlarged print; auditory or hearing techniques; and so on.

3. By using special optical devices, such as magnifiers, spectacle microscopes, and telescopes. These will improve your ability to see detail (read and watch television) but may require you to hold material close to your eyes or see through only a small field of view. The benefits, however, usually far outweigh the limitations if you really want to see.

PREPARING FOR THE APPOINTMENT

It will be helpful to me if you think about specific problems you are having at home, work, or school that are related to your vision. This may include problems with reading, watching television, getting around, playing cards, sewing, knitting, woodworking, or other social and recreational activities. Some of these activities may not be helped by the options available, but we cannot be sure unless you tell us the problems. Think about things you would like to be able to see better. Start to think about your goals. It will be helpful to *write down problem areas*, or have the person reading this write them down for you, along with the goals you hope to attain.

The examination may be lengthy. Schedule your visit around your medications and meals, and select a time when you feel your vision is at its best.

WHAT TO BRING

Bring any glasses or magnifying glasses you are using to the examination. If you have any special materials you want to be able to work with—for example, forms, books, or needlepoint—bring them to the examination as well. This is particularly important for materials you use at work or school and hobbies that you might wish to pursue.

FINALLY

This will be your initial visit. I will probably need to see you several times to ensure you are getting the best prescription for your eyes and that the goals you want to accomplish are attained. A series of visits will also give me time to loan you a device to use at home before prescribing the final one. This added home experience will allow us to design the low vision device that will provide the best performance and greatest comfort.

The best low vision service occurs when you and I form a partnership in which each of us understands your goals and works together to attain them.

2 | Initial Low Vision Examination and Evaluation

As you read through this and subsequent chapters you may want to refer to the low vision care outline below. Just as the flow chart in the introduction is designed to keep you aware of where you are in the global process, this outline is designed to guide your evaluation and follow-up. Please note, under *Modify direction when needed*, that it may be appropriate to change your approach or go through a reality check for you and the patient. Modifying direction or goals may lead to less frustration and more success.

Low Vision Care

Know the outcome: Goal-oriented history
Evaluate and manage: Examination and follow-up
Monitor the outcome:
        In office—SOAPS format for record keeping (Subjective, Objective, Assessment, Plan, Subjective)
        At home—telephone calls to check patient progress, and patient diary
Modify direction when needed:
        Approach—different forms of magnification or minification
        Outcome—reality check, modifying unrealistic goals

This chapter will help you organize a low vision examination; the initial, or consultation, visit is outlined in two parts. The first part covers all the tests and forms needed to conduct the initial examination. The second part explains how this information should be used to form a low vision–device evaluation. These discussions are presented in a clinical, user-friendly manner because there are excellent books in the literature that cover the more extensive and theoretical issues related to the examination. (See the suggested reading list at the end of this chapter.)

CONTENTS

OVERVIEW OF INITIAL EXAMINATION

You should allow approximately 1–1½ hours of face-to-face examination time with a new low vision patient. In addition, allow 15–20 minutes before the actual evaluation for an in-depth history of the patient, to be taken by you or a member of your staff.

All low vision practitioners have their own methods of evaluating patients. The following guideline for the low vision evaluation is exactly that—a guideline. Many factors are intentionally not considered in this discussion. You will have to modify and improvise based on your patient's age, both chronological and developmental, and on any additional impairments or communication disabilities of your patient. Ideally, as you develop your practice and establish a philosophy of care for the visually impaired, you will modify and redesign this guide to reflect your approach.

Before you begin the examination be sure you have received a completed copy of the patient's Brief History (see Form 1.4), which the patient should have received in the information packet before the initial visit. Remember that a formal, in-office history that covers all aspects of the patient's visual life should be taken when the patient is in the office.

Included in the examination form (see Form 2.1) are examples of typical questions. Initially, they can be used verbatim. As you gain experience, you will develop your own phrases to elicit the information. Every item should be explored until you are satisfied that you have enough information to formulate a plan of treatment. The patient's primary and secondary goals will ultimately direct the clinical evaluation. The bulk of time following this in-office history is devoted to examining and evaluating the patient so that you will be able to identify successful methods of resolving the patient's reported visual difficulty.

The initial visit is diagnostic in nature. With the information from the brief history and the formal, in-office history, you will have a feel for the handicapping effect of the patient's vision loss. Your job as a low vision clinician is to minimize this handicap. To do that, you must know and understand the extent and impact of the impairment (vision loss) so you can describe your patient's visual functioning to all those involved in the rehabilitation process, including the patient's family. Following the examination procedures described in this chapter will provide that information. You will demonstrate your expertise and encourage confidence in your abilities by being able to accurately describe your patient's visual functioning. Throughout the examination, think about the magnification, field of view, lighting needs, working distance, contrast needs, and skills necessary to accomplish the goals of the patient.

At the conclusion of the first visit you should

1. Have a specific plan for helping the patient with optical and nonoptical options.
2. Be able to explain the relationship between the disease and the vision-related functional difficulties of the patient.
3. Convince the patient of the need for continued care by the referring doctor.
4. Identify all other community rehabilitation sources appropriate for the patient.

An evaluation of a former patient is slightly different from the evaluation of a new patient. This appointment should revisit the patient's functional and disease concerns. Sometimes a new or existing condition complicates the reason for the patient's initial visit. At this examination you will

- Review the patient's overall medical history and specific visual history.
- Make general observations about the patient's overall well-being.
- Perform tests necessary to determine any functional or disease changes.
- Make recommendations for additional optical and nonoptical changes that may be necessary.
- Encourage the patient to continue to see the referring doctor.
- Re-establish the patient's relationship with any necessary visual rehabilitation services.
- Schedule additional appointments for continued monitoring of the psychophysical effect of the diseased condition of the eye.

This visit typically takes 30–45 minutes.

LOW VISION EXAMINATION

The successful low vision clinician will have the patience demanded by an emotionally fragile pediatric or geriatric patient with an end-stage visual pathology and the ability to interpret the information gathered from a nonverbal, multiply impaired, or cognitively dysfunctional patient with a traumatic brain injury. You should, however, have the same goal for these seriously impaired patients as for more typical patients—that is, obtaining a correction that will provide optimal acuity and enhance visual performance. Patients who are visually impaired, however, encounter the added challenge of learning how to use their new level of sight within the limitations of their disease and the optical properties of the systems that will benefit them. You must be patient in the administration of tests, and you will learn how to develop and modify the testing according to the individual demands of each patient.

The low vision examination begins similarly to a conventional examination—with a complete medical and visual history. However, you will need to add a more complex history or interview regarding your patient's functioning. As with all examinations, problem areas must be identified and specific goals for the outcome of the examination must be established. As in the primary care examination, the low vision examination includes an assessment of acuities, refraction, binocularity, visual fields, contrast sensitivity, eye health, and so forth. This data, however, usually leads to further testing, which will ultimately direct treatment options.

This chapter walks you through a low vision examination, providing insight on the techniques for administering the tests as well as help in interpreting the data collected. If successful, you will move beyond rote administration of these tests to a more sophisticated level of thinking on your own, providing an individualized examination for each of your patients.

First Impression
The examination process begins when the initial appointment is scheduled. Rarely does a patient call simply to make an appointment. Many questions are usually asked. It is therefore important that a member of your staff be knowledgeable about what you do and take the time to answer all of the caller's questions. This usually puts the caller at ease and reduces the patient's anxiety about coming to your office. It also helps to shape the caller's realistic expectations of the low vision process. Most important, it will make the caller feel more at ease when arriving at the office. Nothing is more reassuring than to hear a patient greet your receptionist with "Hi, Paula. I'm so glad to finally meet you." This usually means that your staff did an excellent job during the telephone interview, and the patient has developed an initial comfort level with your office. An incoming positive attitude goes a long way in keeping the patient positive about the vision rehabilitation process.

The initial visit is also a good time for you and your staff to observe the interaction between the patient and family or anyone accompanying the patient. Are the significant others supportive or do they seem removed from the problem? If the family member refuses to sit in the examination room with the patient when invited, what does that mean? It is not always easy to determine who will be supportive of the patient. Sometimes the person you think will not be positive turns out to be the best support imaginable.

Your first impression of the patient's level of independent functioning develops as you watch the intake process at the front desk and in the waiting room. You should be able to learn a lot about the patient even before he or she sits down in the examination chair. However, those impressions can change. Do not set these impressions in stone; over the course of your practice you will note that attitudes often change based on the successful completion of goals.

It may be helpful to make an initial assessment of the patient's demeanor or attitude. Patients can seem depressed, anxious, hyperactive, nervous, or fretful. A short note in the record will remind you of subsequent changes in demeanor as future visits are completed. (The wording of these notes is important because these records may be reviewed by others—for example, lawyers, primary care doctors, third-party payors, and so forth.) It will also remind you of any special considerations required for the patient's follow-up visits. It does help to have a good idea of the patient's personality.

Case History

The case history can take from 20 to 40 minutes to complete. The information collected should provide a good description of the patient and specific goals. It is also important that you feel confident that all proper medical attention has been provided and the functional disabilities reported by the patient are consistent with the systemic condition and your visual findings. The history should be taken in a relaxed setting. The patient needs this time to become comfortable with you and your staff. This is a good time to casually chat with the patient, in addition to seeking specific answers to your questions. This will help the patient to relax. Relaxation encourages trust and may facilitate the evaluation and educational process, which will in turn foster more reasonable patient expectations. The case history should provide enough information to begin thinking about rehabilitation programs and optical and nonoptical options. The rest of the data you explore will revolve around the patient's level of acuity, magnification and lighting needs, and the best format for prescribing a successful device—for example, telescopes, microscopes, magnifiers, telemicroscopes, or electro-optical and nonoptical systems.

Specific questions can be asked as part of the clinical assessment or by sending an in-depth questionnaire for the patient to complete before the appointment. If the latter option is taken, extra time must be allowed for the 20–40% of patients who will not have completed these forms before their appointments. In Chapter 1, we suggest sending a very short questionnaire to the patient. This is an effort to have the patient think about some of the issues that are most important. Think of these questions as the "jumping-off" point for the in-office history.

Medical History/Review of Systems

1. When was your last physical?   Doctor:
2. How did the doctor say your health was?
3. What is your opinion of your health?
4. Do you have any allergies? If so, list here.

Do you or any member of your family have problems with (S = self, F = family):

1. Heart:	S	F	How long?	Medications:
2. Circulation:	S	F	How long?	Medications:
3. Kidney:	S	F	How long?	Medications:
4. Liver:	S	F	How long?	Medications:
5. Lungs:	S	F	How long?	Medications:
6. Skin conditions:	S	F	How long?	Medications:
7. Hypertension:	S	F	How long?	Medications:
8. Neurologic disease:	S	F	How long?	Medications:
9. Endocrine:	S	F	How long?	Medications:
10. Diabetes:	S	F		

   a. How long have you been diabetic?
   b. How is your diabetes controlled?
      1. Diet
      2. Oral medication
      3. Insulin   What type?   Dosage:
   c. How is your glucose monitored?
      1. Urine strip   Average reading:
      2. Glucometer   Average reading:
      3. A_1C (glycosolated hemoglobin)
      4. Physician   How often?
   d. How often do you become hypo/hyperglycemic?
   e. Are you a member of the American Diabetes Association?

11. Gastrointestinal:	S	F	How long?	Medications:
12. Musculoskeletal:	S	F	How long?	Medications:
13. Stroke:	S	F	How long?	Medications:
14. Depression:	S	F	How long?	Medications:
15. Traumatic head injury:	S	F	How long?	Medications:
16. Other:	S	F	How long?	Medications:

Medical History/Review of Systems

A systems review is necessary and can add valuable information related to secondary dysfunctions, physical (motor) problems that may interfere with the handling of devices, mental disorders, strokes, mental deficiencies (e.g., Alzheimer's disease) that may interfere with cognitive responses, and so forth. For some systemic diseases, such as diabetes, self-care and medication administration may become the focus of the low vision examination. A review of systems can be very time consuming, especially if previous medical records are not available. It is important to take notes on this and any other aspect of the history. The more detail you can elicit from the patient, the more thorough the history and the better the base from which you can work. Many third-party payors will not accept checklists but rather require some form of notation to know that the material was in fact discussed.

Visual History

1. How long ago did you first know you had a vision problem?
2. When was your last eye examination?
3. Who was your doctor?
4. Were your eyes dilated?
5. Have you ever had treatment or surgery for your eyes?
6. Are you taking eye medications?
7. Have you had recent changes in your vision?
8. Have you ever had a low vision evaluation?
9. Who was your doctor?
10. What have your doctors told you was the cause of your visual problem? Explain your problem to me.
11. Do you wear glasses now? If so, do they help?
12. How well do you think you see now?
13. Is there any family history of glaucoma, cataract, blindness, or any other eye problem?

Visual History

A visual history is no different than a history taken in a primary eye-care setting with the exception of a potentially more extensive review of various optical and nonoptical devices that may have been previously prescribed. You may also need to go into more detail about previous surgical procedures and medical treatments, as they may affect your ultimate prescriptive considerations.

It is important to know the success of the procedures previously performed and the patient's attitude toward them. As an example, if the patient is still angry at the surgeon who performed laser therapy and feels the procedure was responsible for the present vision loss, this patient may not be able to give complete attention to the low vision process. While you are talking about help, the patient may still be stuck in the "if only" mode. In these situations it sometimes helps to explain previous procedures from an academic perspective. Most procedures are performed correctly, but not all procedures end with positive results. This must be explained carefully to the patient without leaving him or her with the impression that you are "defending" the last doctor. By keeping the explanation educational and encouraging the patient to let you help, you will begin to help move the patient forward.

If a patient has a device or prescription, it is important to determine why the device is or is not being used. If the patient is upset because the last doctor prescribed a pair of glasses that could only be "used up close to the nose," it might not be a good idea to think about starting with a microscopic prescription unless you better explain the microscope, or you may prefer to start with something that allows greater working distance.

This is also a good time to discuss the patient's ocular condition. Does the patient know what the disease is and its implication for further loss of visual function or total vision loss? For example, some patients with macular degeneration still think they are going to become completely blind. With that thought it may be hard to get them involved in a difficult and time-consuming training program. Therefore, it is very important to take the time to describe any disease process in terms that are easy to understand. It will be helpful if you practice these explanations with your staff. You may be amazed at how difficult it can be to explain a disease like diabetes, macular degeneration, glaucoma, retinitis pigmentosa, or others in "lay" terms. If you take time to do this, however, it can significantly improve your relationship with your patient.

Breaking Down Communication Barriers   Some DOs and DON'Ts of communication with the low vision patient are found in the following chart taken from the Second International Conference of Low Vision (February 1988, Los Angeles, CA) [1].

It will solidify your rapport with the patient during this history if you can demonstrate your knowledge of the functional or daily problems precipitated by the disease or treatment process. For example, asking patients with macular degeneration if vision comes and goes or if there is a problem with glare will help to convince them that you understand the functional problems. This may seem basic, but if no other doctor has indicated any knowledge of these functional problems and has ignored the patient's complaints, your ability to describe the disease process will enhance your credibility. Your image as a rehabilitative doctor is developed as you speak. If there is potential for total blindness, the patient should be told in an empathetic way and given an opportunity to prepare for the loss of sight with positive direction toward community as well as family support. In this situation you should have ready the names of outside resources and help to ensure that proper emotional support is available through various social and psychological services. In the case of potential blindness, a carefully penned letter to the attending physician or optometrist is required. The patient's primary care doctor may not have been prepared to handle this delicate issue; the letter should reflect your understanding of the difficulty of the case.

DOs and DON'Ts

DO

Be an open listener, asking questions and clarifying answers to assure understanding.

Look at all available input and respect information from other service providers.

Provide explanations when using vision-related terms.

Allow for misjudgments.

Discuss eye conditions in a way that provides persons with a clearer understanding of the functional implications of these conditions.

Include parents in their child's educational and eye-care programs as often as possible—they are a valuable resource.

Participate in regular meetings with staff to reassess strengths and weaknesses of your particular program and its recommendations for the low vision individual—include input from the low vision person and family members or significant others.

Encourage and actively participate in low vision consumer and professional awareness.

Tell low vision persons where they can learn more about their condition and available services to assist them.

Think before you speak and remain aware of the professional language barriers that you unconsciously help to create and allow to persist.

DON'T

Assume others understand your professional terminology.

Assume all staff and other education, rehabilitation, or community agencies understand your procedures for programming, planning, and implementation.

Speak unfavorably of other service providers.

Make absolute statements.

Tell low vision patients not to worry because they won't go totally blind ... and then walk away.

Refer to the low vision patient in the third person, as if he or she is not there.

Formulate ideas about a low vision patient's abilities, based solely on eye reports and other assessments.

Think of optical aids or devices as the only solution to the visual problems of individuals with low vision.

Use vision-related jargon such as ARM (age-related maculopathy).

Underestimate your role in helping to break down the language barriers in low vision.

Psychosocial History

1. What is your present living situation?
2. Are you able to take care of yourself?
3. What was the last school grade you completed?
4. Do you smoke now?   Y   N
   a.   If yes, how much?
   b.   Smoked for 1 year or more?   Y   N
5. Have you had any rehabilitation training? Do you use assistive devices?
6. In what kind of social or recreational programs are you involved?
7. Who helps with your transportation?
8. Where do you get support? (family, friends, etc.)
9. How do you feel about your vision loss?

Psychosocial History   Psychosocial considerations are complicated and delicate. These interactions require a lot of experience because you will be asking personal and emotionally loaded questions. These questions address issues of family support, financial problems, and general living conditions, which may require community support, social services, or psychological counseling. All of these will be important background when establishing a treatment program. If the necessary support cannot be provided directly or through referrals, the patient may become so involved with locating those services that the low vision treatment program may not be initiated. You should probably ease into these issues until you have developed more experience in understanding the low vision patient's psychosocial problems and how to identify good community support systems. (In some low vision centers, these questions are the responsibility of a social worker involved in the intake process.)

The following information summarizes the work of psychologist Steve Shindell. A review of this information provides some background to help you manage the psychosocial concerns of your low vision patients/clients.

1. *All behavior is purposeful.* That is, there is a reason people act and react the way they do. Simply wishing they were different only tends to cause frustration and anger. The first step in any problem solving should include asking yourself, "What would make this person behave this way?" This could lead to consideration of irrational beliefs, inadequate coping styles, or a disparity in rehabilitation goals.

2. *The client may not be the problem.* In fact, even if the client is, the best solution may not involve him or her. For example, in some agencies there are conflicts concerning the issuance of aids.

Often clients are labeled with pejorative diagnoses, such as *malingering*, because staff members perceive some behaviors as an attempt to obtain equipment that is of no use to the patient. Although it is acknowledged that certain clients fit in this category, what often happens is that clients are given confusing or contradictory information concerning the "rules" of the system and, as a result, attempt to obtain equipment the best way they know of. This equipment may not be necessary but may be desirable for other reasons (e.g., in case their vision deteriorates or because they like the fancy technology). Similarly, we often reinforce passive behavior in certain clients (e.g., clients who become "pets" or who must follow a very structured rehabilitation plan) while attempting to explain the necessity of independence. These iatrogenic effects, or negative impacts caused by the treatment, are inherent in any service structure. Rather than being ignored, they should be examined and diminished whenever possible through staff education, policy changes, and so forth.

3. *Psychosocial rehabilitation is everyone's responsibility.* Teaching a person to effectively interact with the world is as much a part of rehabilitation as teaching long-cane technique. It should not be viewed as an obstacle to treatment but rather as part of the treatment itself. A successful and useful mobility or low vision lesson may focus completely on these factors and still be working on the common goal of rehabilitation—to have clients achieve a high quality of life.

Entry into the Rehabilitation System   Many clients never enter the rehabilitation system because of misperceptions about eligibility or need, lack of information, denial, or depression. In addition, the client's goals are often more limited in scope or more grandiose than the rehabilitation center can provide. Family members may be hesitant to relinquish control over the person with the disability because of fear about issues that may develop if more independence is achieved. Steps can be taken to "go with the client's resistance" by describing rehabilitation in terms consistent with their goals and beliefs. Focusing on information and specific behavioral skills may be less anxiety provoking than presenting rehabilitation in a form that requires immediate and total acceptance of themselves as visually impaired. The process of rehabilitation introduces unfamiliar feelings and situations for the low vision patient.

Following are some recommendations for communicating effectively with patients, according to patient type, provided by Shindell:

1. Clients who know it all (i.e., you can't know—you're not blind)
   - Determine your answer to that question before it is asked

- Remain professional but not dogmatic
- Realize that they have a fragile self-concept that becomes more rigid when provoked

2. Indecisive clients
   - Help them air their reluctance
   - Explore their goals throughout the treatment process
   - Provide support
   - Provide more structure
   - Ask yourself whether you are moving too quickly

3. Clients who say "Yes, but"
   - Do not expect them to "snap out of it"
   - Ask them to provide the solutions
   - Do not feel inadequate
   - Point out how their behavior is keeping them from changing
   - Take control by asking what they see as important to work on and what they have tried that has not worked; concentrate on how to build from their failures

4. Passive clients
   - Do not feel responsible for their silences
   - Have them help make decisions about treatment
   - Ask open-ended questions
   - Encourage them to voice their feelings

5. Hostile clients
   - Do not feel that you have to justify your actions
   - Realize that they are worried about giving up control
   - Recognize when the two of you are in an argument without end
   - Decide what is a successful interaction (e.g., agreeing to disagree)
   - Plan what you say before saying it
   - Tell them how their behavior is influencing how you feel
   - Vent your anger in positive ways
   - Take frequent breaks
   - Recognize and encourage change

6. Manipulative clients
   - Examine what would motivate the patient to behave this way (e.g., the system itself)
   - Be honest and specific in your answers
   - Make sure everyone on the team communicates to prevent staff splitting
   - Control your anger

7. Complaining clients
   - Recognize their need to complain
   - Do not feel guilty
   - Do not get too angry to communicate

- Recognize their feelings while helping them develop good coping strategies

8. Clients who deny their disability
   - Determine what is behind this belief
   - Decide whether this is really impeding progress
   - Allow for compromise (e.g., even though we disagree about the future, what is a problem for you right now?)
   - Structure their doctor-shopping so that they feel comfortable getting your opinion before investing time and money
   - Be honest without destroying the relationship
   - Ask them what they feel life would be like if they were more visually impaired

9. Noncompliant clients
   - Confirm that your examination was accurate
   - Make sure they understand the concept of low vision and what to do
   - Ask how you can work together to change the program to increase their participation
   - Make sure the assignments are not too anxiety provoking or confusing
   - Examine possible positive (e.g., money, attention, escape) and negative effects (e.g., more responsibility, fewer benefits) the client associates with a change in vision. Consider the possibility of them returning at a later date when other factors (e.g., litigation or family issues) are not affecting them
   - Control your anger

Task Analysis

Task analysis is the point at which the history begins to differ from that of a conventional medical or optometric history. You will now pursue a more in-depth look at the handicapping effects or morbidity of the disease process. These questions are fairly standard in a general low vision practice. Their significance is that they require the patient to think about each of the concerns raised and decide how important they are. This functional review should lead to some specific goals for the patient. As these questions are answered and discussed, patients begin to understand that this rehabilitation process is problem oriented and not curative. This review also helps the patient to understand that the options being considered are for specific tasks and often multiple prescriptions are needed for different activities. This may also be a good time to briefly describe a low vision device. Systems like magnifiers, microscopes, and telescopes can be introduced but not necessarily used. A brief explanation of the basic issues of magnification can support the use of these systems. You will repeat a number of these concepts throughout the course of the evaluation but because repetition is the basis for memory, especially in this psychosocially fragile population, now is an excellent time to start. One of the simplest ways to describe the concept of magnification is to explain relative size and distance magnification. You can do this by explaining that there are two ways to view an object. The first way is to simply increase the size of the object until it is recognizable (relative size magnification); the second is to move closer to the object until it appears to be larger and then focus for that specific distance (relative distance magnification). You should rehearse the explanation of this concept of relative size and relative distance magnification until you can easily explain it with confidence to an elementary student.

Mobility (Travel) History

1. Can you see well enough to get around outdoors?
2. Do you drive?
3. Do you have mobility aids—for example, a cane or a guide dog?
4. Do you have glasses or optical devices that help you get around?
5. Do you have difficulty getting around indoors?
6. Do you tend to trip over low objects, such as curbs or steps?
7. Do you tend to bump into objects at eye level?
8. Do you bump one side of your body more than the other?

Mobility History   When asking questions about independent travel, you should try to uncover whether the patient is suffering from specific mobility problems. You may need to decide whether a mobility evaluation is required. The mobility history also provides some idea of the individual's level of independence. A patient who is still traveling by foot, car, or public transportation may have a positive attitude and a strong desire to use remaining vision to maintain a normal lifestyle. A patient who reports bumping into or tripping over things may be experiencing peripheral vision field loss. Further questioning, observation, and testing can substantiate this suspicion.

Treat the issue of driving with care. If you introduce the topic, the patient may focus on this issue alone and decrease concentration on other distance or near activities for which success can be enjoyed. If your patient asks if driving is allowed, the answer should be put off until after the examination, explaining that further tests are needed before an answer can be given. This is a very emotional issue for any patient. You will gain experience in addressing the goal of driving as you evaluate more patients. In the beginning of your low vision career, it is best to try to put this off until later in the low vision process, especially after some success has been achieved with other distance or near devices and a more rational discussion can be held. If you immediately say no to the patient, you may never have the opportunity to try any other type of device or activity that would give the patient the functional improvements these devices can offer. Most important, learn the rules about driving in your state and in surrounding states.

Distance Vision History

                                          At what distance?   With what device?

1. Are you able to see
   a. Billboards?
   b. Labels?
   c. Faces?
2. Do you attend movies?
3. Do you watch TV?
   If so, what is the screen size?
4. Do you have problems recognizing colors? If so, please explain.

Distance Vision History   Questions about distance viewing are a continuation of the independent travel questions. One of the most common complaints people have regarding vision loss is the inability to see faces of friends in social situations, in stores, or on the street. Other than telescopes, filters, and some electro-optical systems, there is really no good solution to this problem. Sometimes these optical devices are not accepted by individuals as a solution because, for example, they are cosmetically unappealing or the field of view is too small. Treating distance vision problems is another challenging area that is better approached after you have established a rapport with the patient and experienced success helping patients to perform near tasks.

Television viewing is an excellent way to demonstrate relative distance or approach magnification. If possible, have a television available during this questioning so you can demonstrate the improvement of television viewing by moving a few feet from the screen and looking off to one side (to demonstrate eccentric viewing). Later you will compare this type of viewing to that done through a telescope or electro-optical system. This often encourages or motivates your patient to explore relative distance magnification at home. For those who accompany the patient during the examination, it may also be encouraging to note that by modifying the environment the patient can achieve some visual success. With television viewing, it is also important to remind the individuals who accompany the patient that a 35-in. screen or rear projection screen is not always best for the patient. Bigger is not always better. Some patients may be better off using an 11- or 19-in. television on a table approximately 2 ft from their face. The smaller set (particularly high-density imagery) may provide much better contrast and visibility.

Activities of Daily Living

Because of your vision loss, do you have difficulty

- Doing your housework?
- Seeing to cook?
- Seeing stove dials?
- Seeing the flame on the stove?
- Seeing food on your plate?
- Seeing the number pad on the telephone?
- Seeing to groom yourself?

Activities of Daily Living The questions about activities of daily living (ADL) can supply a lot of information. Not only do these questions determine whether a task can be done and its importance to the patient, but, taken as a whole, the complete set of questions also provides an indication of the patient's level of daily activity. Does the patient try to stay active or is the patient losing motivation and becoming depressed? An active person usually has more goals, is easier to work with, and enjoys the fruits of success. Patients who are "sitting around the house being blind" may need extra care. It is important that a goal is established for these patients, hopefully one about which they are truly excited. This may not be easy to ascertain with these patients, as most simply agree with anything you say and are agreeable to any goal you suggest. This person is usually the one who is looking for a miracle cure and who needs to hear that technology cannot provide such a cure. Even if previous clinicians have given these explanations, this is a good time to repeat them.

Many problems identified in this section of questioning may be remedied by home training with a rehabilitation teacher or other rehabilitation professional. There are many effective optical and nonoptical solutions to problems with ADL. You should be aware of these independent living devices as well as community resources for obtaining them.

Near Vision History The next series of questions pertains to the patient's ability to perform a variety of near point tasks. This is probably the most important part of the functional history because the greatest amount of success will involve solutions to near point problems. Reading is usually the most straightforward issue to approach optically and the one most reported as a priority. It is mandatory, however, that you determine exactly what the patient wants to read, for how long, and even if that person can read. Some say they want

---

Near Vision History

At What Distance?   With What Device?

1. Do you read print?
2. Can you read
   a. Newspaper headlines?
   b. Large print?
   c. Textbooks?
   d. Typeset print?
   e. Magazines?
   f. Newspaper?
   g. Telephone books?
3. How much reading do you do now?
4. What size print do you use most?
5. What kind of light do you use for reading?
6. Did you read more before your vision loss?
7. Do you want to read more than you presently do?

---

to read, some have forgotten how, and others say they want to read but may actually mean they want to see like they did before the eye problem occurred. This is a good time to assure the patient that reading is an acceptable goal with a good prognosis, as long as the patient is willing to consider reading as a task that may occur even as close as half an inch from the eyes.

During this discussion, you may want to take the hands of your patient and move them to this close distance. If the patient responds by saying, "whatever it takes," that is a good sign. This patient may change that attitude but at least the initial willingness to try is there. If the response is "I can't read at this distance" or "Are you crazy?" you may want to think about a different approach to reading. You may want to explain that this close distance is only one scenario. You may also consider starting with a more challenging system, such as a telemicroscope for reading with a longer working distance, a hand or stand magnifier, or an electro-optical system. These latter systems generally provide a more comfortable working distance with good contrast and high magnification. If the patient becomes frustrated with these systems, a microscope can be reintroduced and the hands moved to the closer working distance, and before the patient realizes it, the text is clear, the field is larger, and reading is more readily appreciated. Make sure the difference between recreational reading (i.e., reading a book) and necessary reading (i.e., reading bills) is clarified. Reading your mail, bills, and receipts and other short-term identification tasks are more basic to your survival and independence than is reading a book or magazine for leisure. Each may require a separate device.

Illumination

1. Do you see better and are your eyes more comfortable when it is bright and sunny or overcast and cloudy?
2. Do you wear sunglasses?
3. Do you use a visor (hat)?
4. Are you bothered by glare?
5. Do you have more trouble with your vision at night than during the day?
6. Do you use extra light to improve your vision?

Illumination   Proper lighting can be the answer to many vision-related problems. Insufficient lighting is usually the problem, but you must take a careful look to make sure that too much light (i.e., glare) is not being used either. You should get a good description of the light being used in each room of the house. Many older patients think a good light is a 100-W bulb in a lamp with a floral lamp shade. Remember, many patients have been helped with the prescription of a hooded, flex-arm, or gooseneck lamp and a +4.00 D add. Time should be taken to explain what a good light source is. Describe the difference between illumination and glare and the importance, for example, of a hooded lamp for maximum illumination and minimum glare. Make sure the complaints of photophobia are more than just normal reactions to going outside or being in brightly illuminated areas.

Work and School   In the section of other vision-related problems, your patient is given the opportunity to have a more open discussion about functioning. You should concentrate on your patient's ability to perform at home, in school, at work, or at recreational activities. These discussions provide a greater opportunity to discover areas of difficulty that may be managed with low vision devices and for which the patient will be highly motivated to succeed.

Hobbies can be very good goals because they provide motivation. However, most hobbies are at intermediate distances (i.e., 8–16 in.) from the eyes, which may require telemicroscopes or electro-optical systems, presenting more of a challenge to the patient. Thinking about relative size may help the patient in maintaining hobby activities. Large-print playing cards, for example, may solve the problem of seeing the cards, but patients may not use them because they feel that other players may get upset having to play with large cards. They generally do not want to seem different.

Primary and Secondary Goals   Two or three major goals that can be addressed in any low vision examination should be established and reviewed. It is acceptable to help your patient prioritize goals based on the necessity and difficulty of the goal desired.

Work and School

1. Are you involved in any of the following activities now or were you involved before your vision loss?
   a. Sewing
   b. Crocheting
   c. Playing cards
   d. Playing a musical instrument
   e. Swimming
   f. Bowling
   g. Bicycling
   h. Typing or computers
   i. Minor repairs
   j. Other
2. Do you have any particular difficulties at school or work because of your vision?
3. Do you have any particular difficulties around the house because of your vision?
4. How do you spend your days?
5. Tell me about some of your major activities.
6. If your vision can be improved with optical devices, are there any special tasks that you would like to be able to do?

Measuring Distant Visual Acuity

Distant visual acuity (VA) measurement is the first test performed on the patient. If administered correctly, it sets the tone for the rest of the examination. Most patients come to you with the belief that they have very little sight remaining. This is usually due to the construction of the VA charts used in the primary care office. Projection charts have variable and, often, lower contrast; are measured for 20 ft; may not be well calibrated; and, most important, do not accurately measure acuity between 20/100 and 20/400. Often the 20/200 optotype is the last or second to last if a 20/400 letter exists. Patients interpret this as an indication that their vision loss is so severe that they are one or two lines away from being totally blind. It is psychologically important to have the patient respond successfully to the optotypes on the chart for this first test. The more optotypes read, the more positive the patient's outlook about the amount of vision remaining and the prognosis for successful low vision intervention. Watching a patient read several lines on a low vision chart can be as exciting for those accompanying the patient as it is for the patient: All now know there is substantial vision remaining. A reminder must be given to those accompanying the patient, however, to reinforce that the patient does have a visual impairment and has not been malingering. This may prompt the patient to ask why the primary care doctor could not measure what you are measuring. In the patient's mind, one acuity is right and the other is wrong. It is important to explain that the acuity measured with low vision charts is performed with higher-contrast optotypes, has more lines to measure, and may have been measured with eccentric viewing. Therefore, both acuities are correct. (This explanation may also need to be repeated to other caretakers who have multiple reports about the patient. They usually want to know which acuity is "right.")

The Designs for Vision distant number chart (Ronkonkoma, NY) is the gold standard (Figure 2.1). This chart allows you to obtain a response from a patient with acuities as low as 20/7,000 (i.e., $2/700 \times 10/10 = 20/7,000$). Although this is not a level of acuity typically seen in a general low vision practice, it demonstrates the flexibility of the chart. The chart actually has optotypes from 10- to 700-ft numbers. It is not uncommon for a patient to proclaim that this is the first time in years that more than one line on the chart could be seen. This kind of response gets you off to a good start with the patient and gives the patient confidence in your clinical skills. These are important ingredients for a successful rehabilitation program.

Distance acuity testing is initially performed at 10 ft. This test distance doubles the number of lines the patient can attempt on a standard chart, decreases the figure-ground or background confusion, allows for better lighting and less glare, and generally elicits a more positive response from the patient.

When using the distant number chart, the largest 7 or 700-ft number should be presented first at the 10-ft distance. You can even encourage the patient to look or find the 7 on the chart you are holding. Watching the patient scan for the 7 may be the first indication of field loss problems, the need for severe eccentric viewing positions, or null points for nystagmus. You can take this opportunity to ask the patient if the 7 is any clearer when the patient looks above or below the 7. If the answer is yes, discussion of eccentric viewing may be introduced. You have just demonstrated an eccentric viewing position to the patient. Another method to demonstrate eccentric viewing is to hold two different charts a few feet apart (Figure 2.2). Because the patient is trying to view centrally, when one target is fixated, the other will appear in the periphery. In this way eccentric acuities can also be obtained as the patient glances from chart to chart. You can experiment with chart separations and locations to determine whether an optimum eccentric viewing position exists. Once the patient is aware of "looking around the blind spot," there is an almost immediate improvement in functional vision. If the patient says that looking to the side and above or below something helps him or her to see clearly, you know eccentric viewing has already been established. It is helpful, therefore, to determine whether the patient can describe eccentric viewing. This information will help

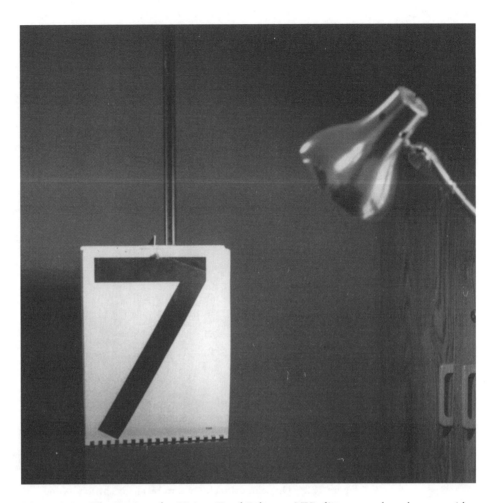

Figure 2.1. The Designs for Vision (Ronkonkoma, NY) distant number chart provides acuity measurements from 10- to 700-ft numbers. This allows the clinician to make a positive measurement of a patient's acuity from 20/7,000 (2/700) to 20/20 (10/10). It is the one way to measure distant acuity in a new low vision patient that will provide a positive start to the examination and goes a long way toward convincing patients they have a lot of vision left rather than dwelling on what they have lost. Proper incandescent, glare-free lighting is important to the acuity measurement regardless of the chart used.

you later in the examination, especially if your patient views to the right (a situation that may interfere with reading and writing).

If the patient reports that the 7 cannot be seen, a severe acuity or field loss may be indicated. If you are observing the patient during this test, it should not be too difficult to determine this. The next step is to bring the chart into a 5-ft test distance. This will increase the range of the chart from 10/700 (20/1,400) to 5/700 (20/2,800). This range allows most individuals with some form perception to respond, or, if the scanning necessary to find the 7 is difficult, may indicate that there is a severe field constriction. Remember that the chart can easily be moved to 2 ft, and an acuity of 2/700 (20/7,000)

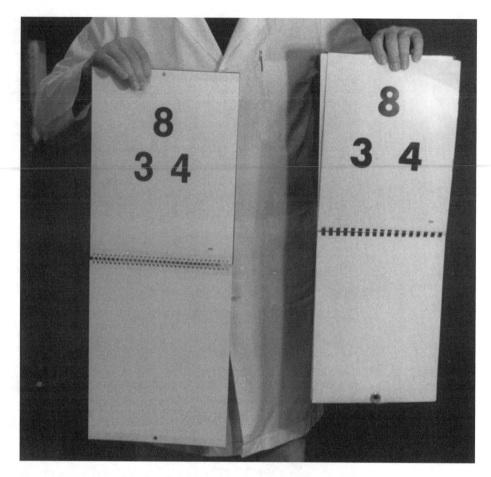

Figure 2.2. One clinical technique to teach eccentric viewing during the acuity test is to use two charts. Have the patient look to the chart on the left and report whether the numbers on the right become more visible. The chart on the left can be shifted more to the left or moved up and down until an optimum viewing (eccentric viewing) position is found. This is a good way to demonstrate eccentric viewing to a patient.

can be recorded. A 2-ft test distance is still a distant acuity measurement for this patient.

If the 7 is successfully identified and eccentric viewing demonstrated, start presenting consecutively smaller optotypes. You should encourage guessing by the patient, encouraging eye movements as necessary to see the numbers. As the numbers get smaller, eccentric viewing, nystagmus, and overall posture may change dramatically as the patient tries to see. It is important to observe this. You may also see a change when there is a transition from single numbers on a page to multiple numbers or lines. During the examination, make note of the following questions:

- Did the patient pick up on the added optotypes?
- Does the patient always miss the numbers on the right or upper numbers?

- Does the patient skip lines or skip from one line to the next and back?

This information is valuable and may describe the position of the field loss, the lack of good fixation, or both. For example, if the patient misses numbers on the right side of the page, tell the patient there are more numbers to the right of the last number identified, and instruct the patient to see if those numbers can be located. An important part of good functional vision skills is awareness of central or peripheral field loss and compensation with good eye movement strategies.

Acuity is recorded as usual (5/20, 10/40, 20/80, etc.). It is often a good idea to indicate in the record that these are low vision acuities and should not be used in the determination of legal blindness. If there is a question about legal blindness, you should test the patient at 20 ft with central viewing on a projected Snellen chart. Often, these more standard measurements are required for legal, social, or eligibility purposes. For example, with the low vision chart, an acuity of 10/60 is measured. This acuity is equivalent to 20/120. However, on the standard projection chart, there are no lines between 20/100 and 20/200. Therefore, this patient will not be able to read the 20/100 and will read the next line, or 20/200, and qualify as legally blind. The issue of legal blindness can be a little more difficult if the low vision acuity measured is 10/50. (The patient may still have a projected acuity of 20/200.)

You need to weigh these measurements with the characteristics of the low vision chart's high-contrast, single optotypes; better figure-ground; and use of eccentric viewing capability. Under these test conditions, the patient may still qualify for services related to legal blindness. You are responsible for what is written in the file and subsequent reports. It would be devastating for a patient to lose important services just because you did not understand the test parameters of the measurement being made.

For psychological purposes it may be best to start with the better eye and test the other eye after success has been demonstrated. However, it is probably not a significant factor, and sometimes it is good to have the better eye tested last so the next test can be started on a positive note. Unaided and aided acuity should be checked during the first visit. Sometimes the patient is unknowingly wearing a prescription that actually reduces the distance acuity. Some patients feel their glasses do not help when, in fact, they make a big difference; others say they help tremendously when they provide no change in acuity. Extra time spent measuring acuities can help tremendously with gathering functional information.

As mentioned before, the Designs for Vision distant number chart is very good for a positive psychological approach to an acuity test. It does not allow, however, for accurate predictions of changes in acuity with the use of magnification or test distance. For example, as the test distance changes or the chart is viewed through a telescope, different optotypes or numbers are seen with different levels of difficulty than were first measured. (One number is on the line when the acuity is taken with glasses; three numbers are on the line with the telescopic acuity measurement.)

There are charts that provide enough optotypes to elicit a positive response from most patients at the 10-ft distance and provide a consistent acuity task from line to line or test distance to test distance. The more commonly used charts are the Bailey-Lovie logMAR (logarithmic minimum angle of resolution) chart (Figure 2.3), Early Treatment Diabetic Retinopathy Study, and University of Waterloo charts. All of these charts have five letters per row and each row has letters of equal difficulty to identify. The spacing between the letters and lines is consistent and based on the size of the letters viewed. The most significant factor regarding these acuity tests is that the size progression of the letters is logarithmic, meaning there is a constant relationship and equivalent acuity measurement for all test distances. Most important, the acuity improvement with a telescope is more predictable because the same task difficulty is required of the patient with the habitual acuity as the acuity taken with the telescope. For example, a 4× telescope provides the same improvement in acuity as moving the chart four times closer. The logMAR chart is also valuable when there is concern about the reliability of the patient's responses. The clinician can be more confident about suspected malingering if the results of the Bailey-Lovie test indicate different acuity levels at two different test distances.

Distance acuity can be recorded in Snellen (foot) or metric (M) notation. In this text the Snellen notation is used for distant acuities. The conversion to M system is listed in Appendix A. The M system is almost always used when discussing near acuity measurements. This way the reader gets some experience with each system and becomes comfortable with both.

Sometimes you will need to measure the acuity of a patient who cannot respond to letters or numbers. In this case there are some good options. A symbol acuity system (Precision Vision, Villa Park, IL) was designed by Dr. Lea Hyvärinen. Symbol optotypes can be used so that the patient can respond directly or match symbols. This creates fewer distractions for the patient and increases the chances that the patient will look at the chart and try to respond. If successful at 5 ft, you can move the chart to 10 ft and compare data for an even more reliable measurement. If the patient cannot name or match the symbol, an estimate of the acuity can be made by having the patient point to the card that you name. You hold one card in each outspread hand and ask the patient to point to a particular symbol.

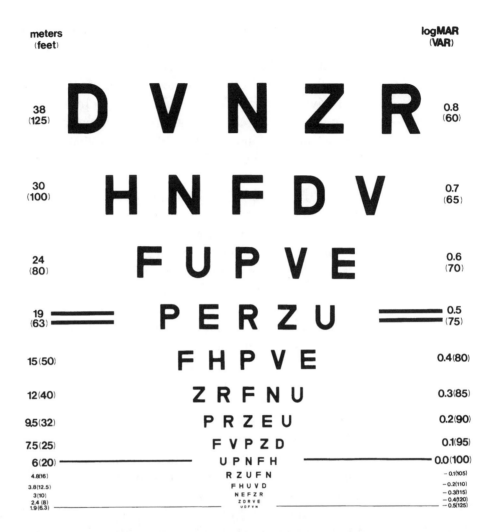

Figure 2.3. A scientific and repeatable measurement of distant acuity for a low vision patient is with one of the logarithmic minimum angle of resolution (logMAR) charts. The Bailey-Lovie logMAR chart shown allows the clinician to vary viewing distance and magnification and still obtain equally difficult acuity task measurements. This is an excellent chart to use for suspected malingering.

Other measures of VA can also be performed. The optokinetic nystagmus drum can be used to predict the presence of functional acuity. A brisk response from 1–3 ft can be interpreted as the potential for some functional vision. A response at 5 ft is an excellent prognosis for visual functioning. A response at a few inches could mean some functional vision is available or that there is only some form perception. However, a positive response or no response may also *not* be significant because there are so many neurologic and pharmacologic influences on this reflexive response.

A response to a light can be of some help in determining if a child or adult has any vision. Occasionally, just observing the patient, especially when favorite toys or food are presented, will give some indication of the presence of functional vision. Sometimes you will have to be creative to establish a baseline measurement, such as "2-in. cookie at 16 in." as the VA for this patient. (See Appendix A for instructions on translating this into a visual acuity.) If a measurement of the level of acuity still cannot be obtained, it is advisable to seek consultation from a clinic or center where formalized preferred retinal locus (PRL) testing can be performed or visual evoked potentials or other electrodiagnostic testing is available. Finally, for more physically and mentally complex children, diagnostic patching can be done to arrive at behavioral visual responses [2].

As with all the acuity measurements, the purpose is to obtain a baseline reading from which future changes in vision or visual functioning can be monitored. The acuity measurement will provide some idea as to the relationship between the patient's disability or vision loss and the patient's report of the handicapping effect of the vision loss. Most of the time, the measured loss and reported loss are consistent. However, you may often find a patient with 20/40 vision who reports an inability to cook, dress, and keep house or a patient with 20/400 acuity who reports still being able to drive safely. Both of these cases show an inconsistency in the measured acuity and the individual's functioning. Patients require special management for both the psychosocial aspects and the magnification treatment of the vision loss.

Acuities should be recorded as the actual test distance, the optotype seen, the type of chart, lighting conditions, and any special ways in which the measurement was made or the patient responded. It is helpful to teachers and other caretakers if you put the 20-ft equivalent in parentheses. A properly recorded acuity would look something like this:

> 10/80 (20/160) room illumination on Designs for Vision distant number chart
> Turns head to the right and misses numbers on right
> Nystagmus decreases in left gaze

You should provide as many descriptive notes as possible about the patient or patient's responses while performing the acuity measurement. Notes should be added about posture, guessing, lighting, eccentric viewing, looking over glasses, pulling glasses down the nose, squinting, shading of the eyes, and so forth. In the above example, it may be better to record an acuity equivalent to 20/200 to maintain the legal blindness status, particularly if this is to be used as a legal document. It may also be appropriate to record the actual equivalent acuity of 20/160 and make a statement on the record that "these are low vision acuities and should not be used in the determination of legal blindness."

When measuring this acuity, if it is apparent that the patient is not eccentrically viewing and will not look above or below the chart, this should be recorded in your descriptive notes. One way to force eccentric viewing is to have the patient look in the direction of the chart. Then quickly move it laterally. For an instant, the number should appear to the patient and then disappear as a saccadic eye movement to the chart is made. For example, the chart can be moved quickly downward or to the right to simulate eccentric viewing upward or to the left. This may be enough to demonstrate to the patient the concept of eccentric viewing and initiate an eccentric viewing response. It is often surprising to the new low vision clinician how many patients have not learned the simple concept of eccentrically viewing targets or "looking around the blind spot."

It is important that the notation of finger count be avoided in recording acuities. It is unnecessary because the patient who can respond to counting fingers can also give a very good response on any of the discussed low vision acuity charts. It is far more accurate to obtain an acuity with a chart than with fingers and it is more reassuring to a patient to be able to read from a chart than to have only enough vision left to see the doctor's fingers at 2 ft. Often "hand motion" acuity measurements are just as invalid. Make sure the level of acuity is really hand movement and that the acuity recorded does not reflect the clinician's failure to use an appropriate chart to make a more accurate measurement.

Distance Acuity and the Low Vision Prescription

The aided and unaided acuity results will inform you of the need for a refraction. If the acuity becomes worse with the present prescription, a complete refraction is in order. If the acuity stays the same or is consistent with the prescription, a simple pinhole or over-refraction may be all that is needed. If the patient does not wear the present prescription and it improves the acuity by three or four lines, you have some other psychosocial matters to consider. With children this often means they do not want to wear glasses. Do not assume that this is the reason, however, as there can be good optical or physiologic reasons for not wearing glasses (e.g., loss of contrast, optical distortions, reduced field of view).

The best corrected distance acuity measurement can be used to determine the magnification needed for a distance device but can also serve as a starting point for the amount of magnification needed for a near device. By taking the denominator of the 20-ft distance acuity and dividing it by the denominator of the target acuity, you will arrive at the magnification needed to perform that task. At distance, a patient with 20/200 acuity who needs 20/50 for distance tasks will need a 4× telescope or electro-optical system (i.e., 200/50 = 4×). If it is determined that this patient needs to see 20/40, then the initial magnification needed would be 5× (i.e., 200/40 = 5×). These are only starting points, however, and should be refined with patient experience and other test results.

Low Vision Refraction

It is important that the acuity loss measured is due to the pathology and not due to a poor refraction or uncorrected refractive error. If retinoscopy shows a bright and fast reflex, a pinhole shows no increase or a decrease in acuity, or subjective responses to lenses reveal no difference, you can feel confident that the measured acuity represents a loss due to the pathology and not an uncorrected refractive error. A trial frame refraction should always be performed.

When a full low vision refraction is indicated, the trial frame is always used with initial reliance on retinoscopy. (Cloudy media, eccentric viewing, nystagmus, reduced acuity, and poor subjective responses all make the low vision refraction more time-consuming but not impossible. Often the low vision refraction elicits different responses than the refraction performed in the primary care setting. Neither refraction is wrong—they are just different.) If needed, retinoscopy can be performed at distances of 40, 20, or even 10 cm (Figure 2.4). This is radical retinoscopy and may give you an indication of the presence of a substantial refractive error for the patient. When a full low vision refraction is indicated, appropriate work distance lenses (+2.50, +5.00, and +10.00 D, respectively) must be used.

When looking at the retinoscopy reflex, you should get into the habit of looking for a reflex equivalent to a ±20.00 D hyperope or myope with −8.00 D of cylinder. If you establish this in your mind before the examination, you will be less likely to miss significant refractive errors. When performing retinoscopy, continue placing stronger lenses in front of the eye until a reflex is seen. A −30.00 D myope will not have a recognizable reflex until you use a −15.00 or −20.00 D lens! Further sources of discussion of techniques for the trial frame refraction are found in the suggested readings.

Even if you cannot see a reflex with radical retinoscopy and ±20.00 D lenses, you should conduct a trial frame subjective. Ask the patient to view the line above the threshold measurement on the acuity chart. Plus and minus lenses of 2.00, 5.00, 10.00, and 20.00 D are presented to the patient and a subjective response regarding visual improvement is requested. Cylinder can be checked in each major meridian with a −4.00 and −8.00 D trial frame cylinder lens. Cylindrical lenses can also be put in the trial frame and the patient asked to rotate the lenses to see if there is any position in which the

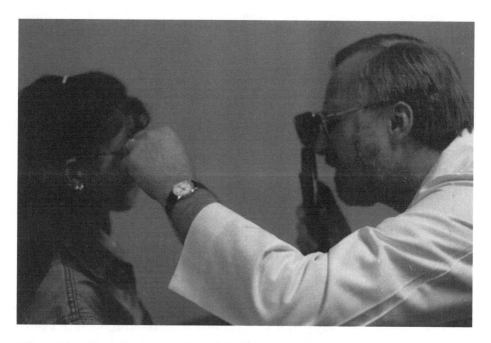

Figure 2.4. The retinoscopic reflex of the low vision patient is often difficult to see. To obtain a better or brighter reflex, the clinician can work at reduced viewing distances and use appropriate compensating lenses. In this figure, the clinician is working at 25 cm using a +4.00 D neutralizing lens. If necessary, a 10-cm work distance with a +10.00 D compensating lens can be used to help define a refractive error reflex.

lenses render the acuity chart clearer. One diopter Jackson cross cylinders are available for a subjective refraction for astigmatism. Stenopaic slits can be used to determine the presence of a cylindrical correction. Remember that in all the subjective responses, it may take a 5.00 D change to elicit a response from the patient because of depressed sensitivity. A keratometer can be used (even on patients with nystagmus) to detect the presence of astigmatism. In patients with nystagmus, it helps to keep both eyes open and to try to put the eye in the null point position in the keratometer. It may sometimes help to blur the eye not being tested as a method of decreasing nystagmus.

Refraction and the Low Vision Prescription

Always check the distance acuity when you finish the refraction. You may have found a new prescription that seems to improve the acuity by two lines but when you recheck the acuity with the old glasses it is also improved. The improvement may be that the patient is using eccentric viewing or is simply relaxed and giving better responses. The main information determined from this procedure is whether the refractive error alone needs to be changed or incorporated into the low vision prescription. This will often dictate the design of the system to be prescribed, especially if cylinder is involved. A single-cut aspheric microscope can be used if there is no subjective difference with a cylinder. However, if 8.00 D of cylinder is required, a doublet microscope, for example, will be required. If the refractive error does not improve acuity through a telescope, have the patient remove the glasses when looking through the telescope. The decreased vertex distance without the glasses will increase the field of view through the telescope and may give enough field to help improve the patient's functional sight.

Contrast Sensitivity Testing

Two patients with the same distance acuity can function quite differently. You might assume this difference is due to the personality of the patient, with one having a stronger personality and desire to function normally. The difference, however, may be explained as real differences in vision loss that can be measured by contrast sensitivity tests. The typical measurement of contrast sensitivity is with the Vistech 6500 contrast test (Dayton, OH) or CS Vector Vision Chart (Precision Vision, Villa Park, IL). These charts measure high-, medium-, and low-frequency losses of contrast and are more diagnostic than others on the market and can be very valuable in determining a plan of care for your patient. With low vision patients, this test is generally performed at 1 m to ensure a good response. For conventional patients the test is usually performed at 3 m, so the acuity cutoff will be three times greater (the 20/20 cutoff is actually a 20/60 acuity cutoff, etc.).

High-frequency losses mostly affect near point tasks involving detail. A high-frequency loss usually indicates the need for good lighting. (Halogen or xenon and other special lighting may be considered.) Mid-frequency losses are more involved with tasks related to walking and mobility. Curbs, potholes, and steps are more of a problem when there is a mid-frequency loss. Low-frequency losses are related to viewing large objects such as buildings, cars, and people. Obviously, this is an oversimplification because most ADL tasks require all three contrast levels. For example, perception of low-frequency wavelengths is needed to see the body of a person, perception of medium-frequency wavelengths assists with seeing eyebrows and the types of garments worn, and perception of high-frequency wavelengths is needed to see detail such as eyes, jewelry, and facial expressions. However, knowing where the contrast sensitivity function loss is will enable you to explain many of the patient's behaviors and responses. If there is an overall depression of the contrast sensitivity curve, special management is often required. In this case, lighting is as important as magnification. Telescopes may not be recommended because they reduce light. Doublet lenses or other specially designed lenses should be prescribed because they reduce light loss and enhance contrast, resulting in better performance for the patient.

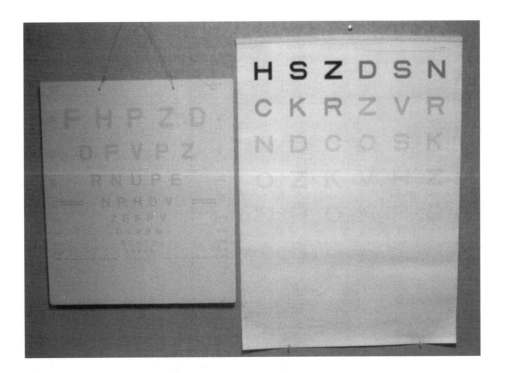

Figure 2.5. Contrast sensitivity testing for the low vision patient is important. The figure shows two charts that can provide quick clinical information about the presence of significant contrast sensitivity problems to be addressed in the design of an optical aid. The Pelli-Robson chart (on the reader's right) is presented at 1 m, and the patient is asked to read as far down the chart as possible. Reading only the top two lines indicates a severe contrast problem, probably overall depression. If the third and fourth lines are read, the problem is a modest loss, and normal lighting concerns should be addressed. With the Bailey chart (on the reader's left) the reduced contrast side of the chart is shown. If the patient loses two lines of acuity or more from the high-contrast measurement (on the other side of the chart), a contrast sensitivity problem can be considered in designing a treatment option or training program.

Occasionally there is not enough time to perform a formal, lengthy contrast sensitivity test, yet information on contrast sensitivity is still needed. Two other tests can provide some basic information on contrast sensitivity concerns. The Bailey Hi-Low Contrast Acuity chart (University of California, Berkeley, College of Optometry, Berkeley, CA) and the Pelli-Robson contrast sensitivity test (Clement Clark, Columbia, OH) are reliable screens for the presence of contrast sensitivity problems (Figure 2.5). If the patient drops two lines or more in acuity when going from the high-contrast side of the Bailey chart to the low-contrast side, a contrast problem is indicated, as it is if the patient can only read the first two lines on the Pelli-Robson chart at 1 m. These two tests are not as diagnostic as the Vistech or Vector Vision tests but are very practical to administer in terms of time and cost. They can indicate a contrast sensitivity problem and the need to address issues of lighting, contrast, filters, and lens design in the determination of an appropriate low vision prescription.

Contrast Sensitivity and the Low Vision Prescription

In general, poor contrast sensitivity indicates that the clinician should give more attention to glare control, contrast of materials being viewed, and illumination. These factors will often be as important to the success of the prescription as the magnification. In fact, you will encounter patients who are doing poorly with a 3× microscope until halogen lighting is added, thereby allowing maximum performance. Without the lighting, 5× magnification may be needed to read the same print size with less proficiency. Do not deny your patients optimum visual performance by neglecting contrast sensitivity testing.

Measuring Near Visual Acuity

The major concern or goal of most of your patients will involve near tasks. Reading is the specific goal of most patients. Therefore, you must measure near acuity. There are numerous charts available with single letters and numbers; multiple letters and numbers; and words, phrases, and sentences with varying levels of difficulty. A suggested starting point is a chart with single letters or numbers. This type of chart will be easiest for the patient to see and elicit the most positive response (similar to the Designs for Vision distant number chart). In fact, when examining your first few patients, it is suggested that the Lighthouse Near Acuity Chart (New York, NY) be used (Figure 2.6). This test chart will draw positive responses and provide a starting point for near point magnification. Initially, you should follow the instructions and present this chart at 40 cm (with the appropriate near lens). As you gain experience, the chart can be handed to the patient with instructions to read as far down the chart as possible. This adds some information to the test results because it allows the patient to set the work distance. If the chart is held at 13 or 16 in. (33–40 cm) and is not moved any closer to attempt to get better acuity when the end point is reached, the patient will need encouragement to read at closer distances. You should consider starting with home training to teach the patient to be comfortable with a closer work distance or lower power devices and large print. If, on the other hand, the patient pulls the material to 8 in. (20 cm) and struggles to read the chart, you can start the prescriptive process by providing the patient with a +5.00 D add for the 20-cm work distance. Often this will result in a significant improvement in acuity and can be an initial add prescribed for daily wear, possibly in addition to a microscopic add for reading small print.

When you initially hand the chart to your patient, the distance the chart is held for the acuity test can be quite revealing as to the approach to magnification you may want to take. It may help you determine the type of device with which you will begin. As an example, a 4× stand or hand-held magnifier will result in better success

THE LIGHTHOUSE NEAR ACUITY TEST

DESIGNED WITH SLOAN LETTERS FOR
TESTING SUBNORMAL VISION AT 40 CM 16 INCHES

PRINT SIZE IN METERS	ACUITY AT 40 CM IN CM			DISTANT EQUIVALENT	DIOPTERS OF ADD FOR AVERAGE PRINT (1M, J #5, 9 Pt.)
16M	40/1600	R K	C S	5/200	40D
13M	40/1300	Z H	D O	5/160	32D
12M	40/1200	D K	H N	10/300	28D
10M	40/1000	D S	V N	10/250	24D
8M	40/800	R H	Z C	10/200 20/400	20D
6M	40/600	K O	N H	20/300	16D
5M	40/500	H N O	R C V	20/250	12D
4M	40/400	C Z H	S D K	20/200	10D
3M	40/300	V R N H Z	D C S K O	20/150	8D
2.5M	40/250	H N O R C	Z S V D K	20/125	6D
2M	40/200	N R C Z H	O V S D K	20/100	5D
1.6M	40/160	D H Z V K	R C O S N	20/80	4D
1.2M	40/120	R N H S O	K D C Z V	20/60	3D
1M	40/100	V R N H Z	D C K S O	20/50	2.5D
.8M	40/80	S O C Z N	H R V D K	20/40	2D
.5M	40/50	[illegible]	[illegible]	20/25	1D

Near vision is tested at 40 cm with best distance correction. If accommodation is insufficient add +2.50.

For visions less than 5/200, test at 20 cm and add +5.00.

"Diopters of add" are an approximation based on reciprocal of visual acuity.

LHNV-1

THE LIGHTHOUSE LOW VISION SERVICE 111 E. 59th St. NEW YORK, N.Y. 10022

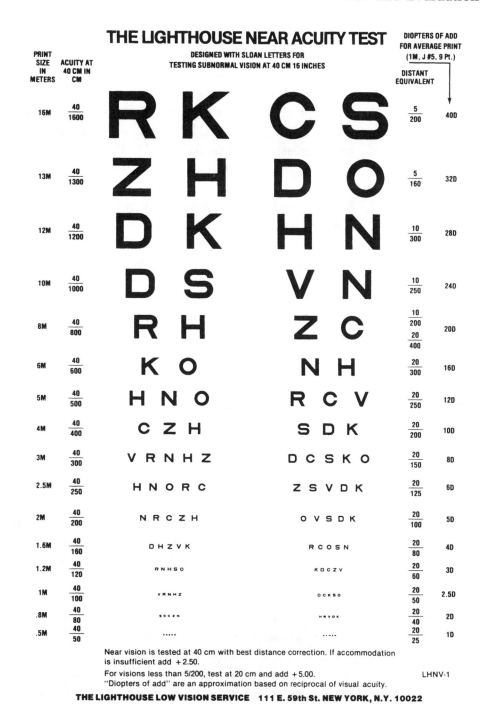

Figure 2.6. The Lighthouse Near Acuity Test provides an excellent and easily administered acuity test for the low vision patient. It is designed in the M system, noted on the right column to help clinicians determine the appropriate lens to start magnification assessment for each patient. It is a great way for new or inexperienced clinicians to ensure success with the demonstration of the first near point prescription. (Reproduced courtesy of The Lighthouse Low Vision Service.)

for a patient who wants to read at 13 in. (33 cm) than a 4× full-field microscope where the material will have to be held at less than 3 in. (6.6 cm) from the eyes.

The near acuity should be taken with and without the habitual prescription used by the patient for near point activities.

In addition to a single optotype near acuity, you should obtain an acuity measurement using a card with sentences or paragraphs. This will give you a second measurement of acuity, an informal assessment of reading ability, and a better base measurement to determine magnification needs when the objective is to read. When measuring near acuities, a very important observation to make is the difference between reading paragraphs or sentences and seeing single letters or numbers on a chart. If this difference in measured acuity is two lines or more (e.g., 2 M with single letters and 4 M with paragraphs), you may consider the vision problem to be more oculomotor in nature rather than just a matter of magnification (sensory loss). The inability to read paragraph material the size of single letter material may indicate a problem with contour interaction, contrast, poor fixation, eccentric viewing, distortion, or the inability to read. A big difference between paragraph acuity and single optotype acuity directs you to address the oculomotor aspect of fixations as a precursor to providing the patient with a magnifier. This patient may report that print swims by or words disappear. The patient may say that things "flash on and off," words may be read wrong, lines and words in a sentence may be skipped, and so forth. Your patient may report the functional problems of being unable to hold fixation at the new preferred retinal locus or eccentric viewing point. It may be helpful to initiate an eccentric-viewing training program before prescribing a low vision reading device. You can initiate a simple home exercise program using a clipboard, stand magnifier, and training exercises that will improve eccentric fixation skills, help the patient become comfortable with a closer work distance, and eliminate frustration (Figure 2.7).

A typoscope (reading slit) should also be demonstrated when measuring near acuities. A typoscope is a small black card with a rectangular window cut out of it. If the typoscope improves the patient's acuity, especially with paragraph acuity, the patient may have an eccentric viewing problem or this patient may require high contrast. Eccentric eye movements are easier to control when the patient is presented with one line of print at a time. The black background of the card also provides enhanced contrast. This is just another way to measure the patient's functional vision and to better describe the patient's ability to perform visually. Figure 2.8 shows a typoscope being used with a Hoeft acuity card.

When recording the near acuity, it is important to note the test distance. This is often more important than the actual size of the letter because it dictates the magnification and indicates the patient's

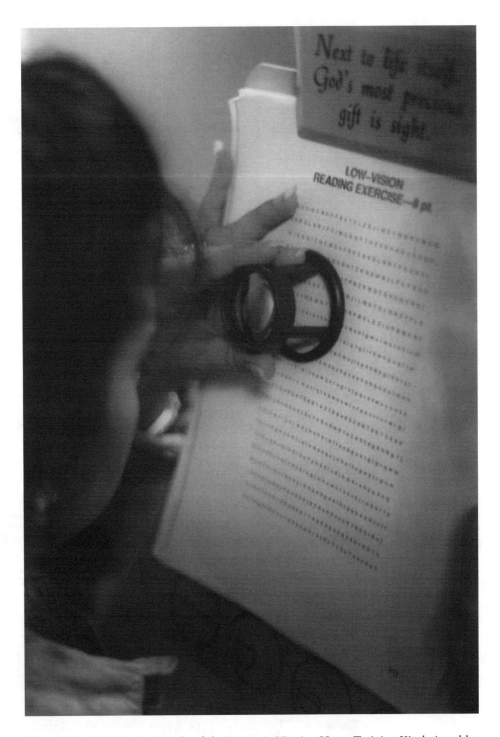

Figure 2.7. This is an example of the Eccentric Viewing Home Training Kit designed by Dr. Randall Jose. It is available through Spalding Magnifiers (Houston, TX, and Mattingly International, Escondido, CA). The kit is an effective way to get patients involved in eccentric viewing training without expensive equipment or multiple office visits. (See also R Jose. A home training kit for eccentric viewing. J Vis Rehabil 1994;9[2]:4.)

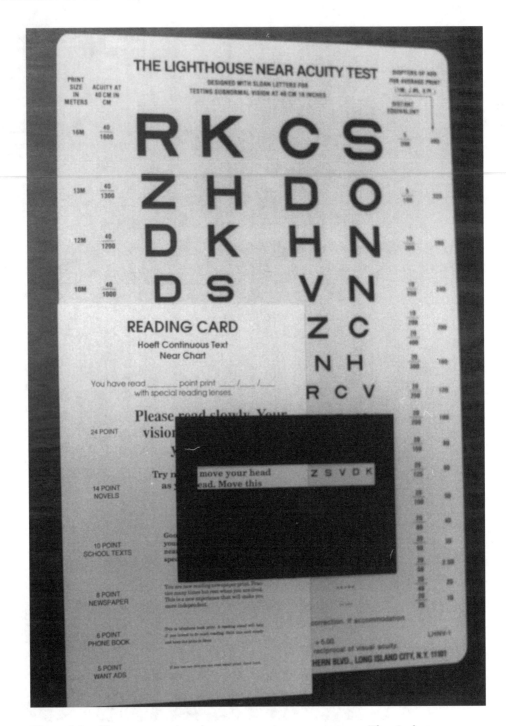

Figure 2.8. There are two important near acuity measurements. The single optotype as shown in Figure 2.6 provides information as to the potential or optimum acuity. The paragraph acuity measurement not only provides information about size resolution but also detects problems in reading skills, tracking skills, and eccentric viewing skills. The Hoeft card shown here is a good paragraph acuity card because it provides good optotypes and leaves patients with a positive message about their vision. It is being used with a typoscope. Both charts should be used in the routine low vision evaluation.

preferred work distance. The lighting used for the test must be indicated along with a description of any unusual head postures, eccentric viewing, or areas of the chart that are consistently missed (e.g., last word on the right, middle letters of most words at least five letters long).

As indicated earlier, the best near acuity chart to start with is the Lighthouse Near Acuity Chart. It is designed to be used at 40 cm. If the chart is held at 40 cm, it is easy to convert acuities into magnification using the scale on the right side of the chart. The Snellen acuities on this chart were calculated at a 40-cm work distance. Therefore, magnification is represented by the formula M = D/2.50 D, or every 2.50 D equals 1× magnification. This dioptric value represents the starting point of add that will allow the patient to read 1 M on the chart.

The calculation is straightforward. Take your measurement of acuity at 40 cm. Record in M notation (5 M at 40 cm or 0.4/5 M). Using the 40 cm or 2.50 D reference, multiply 2.5 × 5 (M) for a starting magnification of +12.50 D. If this is too difficult, simply read to the right of the chart and the notation will be 12.00 D. If you choose to perform the test at a different distance, you must modify the diopter multiplier for the new reference distance. This is shown in the chart below for test distances of 40, 33, and 25 cm.

Test Distance:		40 cm	33 cm	25 cm
Magnification:		D/2.5	D/3.0	D/4.0
Patient's Acuity	1 M	2.50 D	3.00 D	4.00 D
	2 M	5.00 D	6.00 D	8.00 D
	3 M	7.50 D	9.00 D	12.00 D
	4 M	10.00 D	12.00 D	16.00 D
	5 M	12.50 D	15.00 D	20.00 D
	6 M	15.00 D	18.00 D	24.00 D
	etc.	Diopter add required to read 1 M print		

A different example illustrates how a different distance will affect magnification. A patient reading 5 M at 33 cm with the best correction in place (i.e., +3.00 D add), will need an initial add of +15.00 D to read 1 M on the chart. Put the +15.00 add (+20.00 D for a +5.00 D hyperope or +10.00 D for a −5.00 D myope) in a trial frame, hold the chart at the focal distance of the add (or approximately 6.5 cm), and the patient should read the 1 M line on the chart.

Another method of determining an initial starting point for near point magnification is to have the patient read the chart at a comfortable distance. Record the M print size and test distance. If the patient reads 5 M at 33 cm and the goal is to read 1 M, you know that 5× magnification is needed. This can be achieved easily by moving the printed material five times closer than the 33-cm test distance. At approximately 6.7 cm (33/5 = 6.7) the patient will see 1 M print if 15.00 D of accommodation can be sustained (100/6.7 = approximately 15.00 D of accommodation). A +15.00 D add will assure the patient's comfortable 1 M vision at the 6.7-cm work distance.

The initial demonstration should use a full-field microscope to help elicit a successful response. The large field of view of the microscope will help with fixation for even those with eccentric viewing or other fixation problems. If the patient quickly reads the 1 M letters, this microscope can become the prescription (loaned) and training can be initiated with this system. It may also be advisable to take a paragraph acuity with the microscope. Successful reading with the system will provide further confidence that this is the best starting prescription for the patient. If only 1.5 or 2 M print is read, the clinician should consider lighting, eccentric viewing, contrast, typoscopes, metamorphopsia, uncorrected refractive error, or the need to adjust the work distance for the lens before increasing the magnification. There is almost always some reason the patient cannot achieve the theoretic result. Try evaluating these other factors before increasing the magnification. With an increase in magnification, the field of view is reduced, the work distance is decreased, and aberrations of the optical system increased. If you note that the patient holds the material at 4 cm with the microscope, instead of the calculated 6.7 cm and reports it is in focus, the patient either has an uncorrected myopic refractive error or is accommodating to get more magnification. A consistent 8-cm work distance with the material in focus is indicative of an uncorrected hyperopic refractive error that should be evaluated. As you can see, there is more to measuring acuity than getting a number. When deciding on a lens to use for the acuity, remember that you work in diopters. Manufacturers may call a lens system a 5× magnification when it is really 4×. You may think you are working with a +20.00 D lens when in fact it is +16.00 D. The poor patient response, therefore, may be due to an incorrect lens and not a poor acuity response.

Amsler Grid Testing

Amsler grid testing can be administered after the refraction or, as outlined here, after the near acuity measurement. The testing should be performed monocularly and binocularly using the lens appropriate to the viewing distance that enables the patient to see the dot in the center of the grid. It is important to record this distance so the actual degree measurement of the scotoma can be calculated or estimated. (If each square at 33 cm equals 1 degree, then, if the patient holds the grid at 11 cm, each square equals 3 degrees.) A central scotoma is known to exist because of the acuity loss; hence, the purpose of this test is not as diagnostic as when used in a primary care setting. In this case the test is used to determine the quality of the patient's central vision or the perimacular area to be used for magnification and eccentric viewing. The goal of the test is to determine functional information rather than disease information, unless you believe the diagnosis is suspect or there may be a change in the status of the disease process. In the functional test, the patient is asked to look at the dot in the middle of the grid. If the patient cannot find the dot, has a lot of head or eye movement, or cannot hold fixation on the dot, the patient probably has not developed a preferred retinal locus and cannot eccentrically view. In this case, the grid with diagonal fixation lines is used and the patient is asked to look where the lines appear to cross in the middle of the chart. You can then plot the extent of the central scotoma. This can be done by asking how many squares are involved or by using a 1-mm target (e.g., a tangent field test target) and actually plotting the scotoma on the grid.

If the patient can fixate the dot eccentrically, the question is asked as to the presence of missing squares (scotoma) or if any of the squares seem distorted (metamorphopsia). In addition to the medical implications of these responses, the size, number, and location of scotomas and the presence of distortion will provide information regarding the patient's ability to use that area of retina for enhancing visual performance. It may be helpful to have the patient indicate the missing or distorted areas with a pointer. The most difficult aspect of administering this test may be using the language that will make it clear to the patient what is required. For some patients, you only need to tell them to "look at the dot and, while looking at the dot, tell me if you notice any missing areas on the grid or if parts of the grid seem distorted." For others, a more basic explanation may be needed, such as, "pretend the chart is a screen door and tell me if there are any holes in the screen. Do any of the boxes on the chart look funny or distorted or do they all look like perfect squares? Or do they look more like barrels than boxes? Do any of the sides of the boxes appear curved or bent?" With practice, you will be able to think of a lot of analogies for this test procedure.

Amsler Grid and the Low Vision Prescription

The measured best corrected acuity will indicate how much magnification is needed to perform a specified task. The Amsler grid, however, will modify that tentative or initial magnification based on the scotomas and measured areas of distortion. Some examples of how the Amsler grid findings will impact on the treatment plan are as follows:

- Referral for continuing medical care may be indicated if new scotomas or additional metamorphopsia are noted on the Amsler grid. It could also mean the patient is getting better at taking the test!
- A scotoma to the right of fixation may create problems for the patient with reading tasks. The print will seem to jump out of nowhere for the patient and localization and tracking skills will be poor, even with correct magnification. If possible, the patient should be taught to move the scotoma to a superior or inferior position (i.e., look above or below the reading material). Occasionally, adding 8.00–10.00 D base-up or base-down to the loaned prescription will facilitate the new eccentric viewing posture.
- A scotoma to the left of fixation (and sometimes inferiorly) will cause confusion and problems with localization (e.g., getting back to the beginning of the line, finding the next line). This should not preclude work with a near point prescription. Reading/line guides, typoscopes, or a finger at the left margin can help the patient.
- A patient reporting metamorphopsia around the fixation area will have difficulty viewing eccentrically because the sensory system will try to maintain an orientation to those functioning cells in the area of distortion. These patients will use a more peripheral retinal area to view but may not be able to sustain this distortion-free area because the motor system will slip back toward the image seen by the more central and distorted area of retina just outside the central scotoma. In this case the patient will need higher contrast targets and more lighting. The experience of the authors indicates that the need for magnification when distortion occurs is approximately twice what would be predicted from the distance or single-letter near acuity.
- A patient reporting a central scotoma (i.e., cannot see the dot) needs further work on eccentric viewing before the prescription of any optical device. A simple home training system that can be used to teach the patient to view eccentrically in a 2- to 3-week period is described in more detail later in this chapter (see Form 2.2). Once the patient has developed steady eccentric viewing, success with optical devices (distance or near) will be greatly enhanced.
- If binocular viewing of the grid shows less distortion or fewer scotomas than either of the monocular findings, you are encouraged to try to maintain binocular viewing for the

patient when prescribing. This is a good indication that there is some "filling in" of the monocular images under binocular viewing, often resulting in a less drastic eccentric viewing position and more comfortable visual performance with optical systems.

Binocular Testing

The majority of visually impaired patients are monocular; approximately 10% are binocular or enjoy simultaneous perception. You need to assess ocular alignment, however, to determine the potential for obtaining and/or sustaining binocularity with the low vision prescription. For many patients, it is psychologically important for both eyes to work, and you may prescribe a lens in front of the poorer eye even though the image is totally suppressed. It is difficult to assess binocular vision in a visually impaired patient, and there are very few tests that can be used to ascertain true binocular status. It is a more realistic goal for the clinician to determine whether the patient can use two eyes at once (we will call this binocular), if the patient suppresses one eye (monocular), if the patient can use each eye independently (biocular), or if a retinal or sensory inhibition exists from the poorer eye when the patient is trying to use the better eye for detailed tasks (retinal rivalry).

Testing may begin with a simple cover test or Hirschberg's test to determine whether there is motor misalignment. If a strabismus exists and the patient does not report diplopia, monocular vision can be presumed. With nystagmus and poor fixation, you may miss a small deviation. Thus, a patient may be totally monocular because of this small deviation and acuity differences between the two eyes, but present with a seemingly aligned and binocular posture. These are also individuals who, when the acuities are similar between the two eyes, may suffer from sensory inhibition or retinal rivalry. The contrast sensitivity test, when performed under binocular viewing, can be a good assessment of binocular vision. If the patient is not aligned and the binocular finding is the same as the better monocular finding, monocular vision can be assumed. If the binocular finding is depressed or worse than the finding in the better eye, you should strongly suspect the presence of sensory inhibition. In this case, the patient may need to be taught to suppress the poorer eye to maintain optimum visual functioning. If the contrast sensitivity function curve or response on binocular viewing is higher or better than with either eye monocularly, summation has occurred. This is a strong indication that you should strive for a binocular low vision prescription.

If alignment is noted, the Worth four-dot test or the red lens test can be used to determine the presence, if any, of sensory fusion. Even a poor response to these tests should encourage you to try to maintain binocular vision for the patient. When performing the Worth four-dot test, remember that central scotomas do exist and may block one of the circles on the test. Make sure the responses make sense. It may help to have the patient move the eyes around to look at the flashlight to see if the configuration of circles changes. Also, the red and green lights may be referred to as other colors. As long as they are consistent, you can accept this as a reliable response. The responses on the Worth four-dot test are probably the strongest indication of whether a biocular prescription may be possible. With acuities better than 20/100 and fairly equal between the two eyes, gross stereopsis may still exist. The patient (with a high add) may be able to respond to the stereo fly, the Wirt circles, or other stereo tests, demonstrating a higher level of binocular involvement. A positive response indicates a need to try to maintain binocular vision with the low vision prescription.

When there is no alignment but the acuity is fairly equal in both eyes, the patient may be able to alternate the use of one eye while suppressing the other. This alternating vision or biocular status can be very advantageous in prescribing low vision devices. This patient can be given a binocular microscope, and when the right eye tires the left eye can take over. This extends the period of time that some patients can comfortably use a device; for others, it simply adds to the confusion. In some situations this type of patient can be prescribed a microscope for one eye and a telescope for the other or a microscope for one and a conventional lens for the other. The two eyes truly function independently.

The concept of retinal rivalry or sensory inhibition in the low vision patient is not well understood and difficult for most clinicians to incorporate into the treatment plan. However, it is a very important consideration for you, especially if you see patients early in the disease process. The problem is best diagnosed when the binocular reading acuities are worse than those of the better eye, when the contrast sensitivity curve is dampened under binocular viewing conditions, or when the patient automatically covers the poorer eye when the threshold is reached in an acuity measurement. This problem often exists when the acuities are reasonably similar, such as 20/40 in one eye and 20/80 in the other. They are enough alike to stimulate fusion but too dissimilar to allow fusion, thus resulting in the sensory inhibition or interference. Sometimes the diagnosis is easy, as the patient will report ghost images or disparate images when trying to read material at threshold. However, the inhibition can also occur when the acuity is 20/80 in one eye and 20/400 in the other. This is especially true if the 20/400 eye was formerly the dominant eye or was the better eye for the first 1–2 years of the disease process. This is difficult to test for, but you will gain experience in finding this sometimes subtle impairment to visual functioning as you evaluate more patients and the symptomatology is better appreciated.

Binocular Testing and the Low Vision Prescription

Use of the testing regimen described in this chapter will result in a diagnosis of the patient as monocular, binocular, biocular, or with sensory inhibition. Each of these can impact on the low vision prescription as follows:

- Prescribing for a monocular patient is straightforward. The clinician prescribes for the better eye. Another consideration is whether there are any psychological issues to the fitting of a monocular device. Some patients need to believe they are still using both eyes because they fear an unused eye will lose all function.
- A binocular patient is a candidate for base-in prism to help sustain a binocular posture for near tasks if the acuities will allow for the prescription. Binocular prescriptions up to +12.00 D are available with prism. Powers beyond +12.00 D are usually not successful as binocular prescriptions, even with prism.

  Binocular vision is aided by maximum acuity, so cylindrical corrections are important to the prescription. Binocularity is also aided by peripheral fusion, so the larger the field of view of the device prescribed, the stronger the stimulus to gain and maintain fusion. Thus, bifocal corrections may not be as successful as prismatic half-eye corrections.
- A patient with biocular vision is rare but a delight to work with. Use the information you have about the patient's visual needs in prescribing for each eye.
- Retinal rivalry or sensory inhibition can be best managed by patching the worse eye. This may only be necessary during the training sessions and loan period until suppression develops and best acuity and visual performance occur with both eyes open. The patient should be prepared for the possibility of having to wear a patch when the low vision prescription is worn and while performing a detailed visual task. This finding is most prevalent in a patient with minimal macular degeneration with, for example, acuities of 20/30 in one eye and 20/50 in the other. This patient is already wearing a +4.00 D add, astutely prescribed by a previous clinician, but reports that the print cannot be read with the lenses; yet 0.5 M on the paragraph chart was read with the 20/30 eye during the examination. It is not until the acuity test is taken under binocular viewing that you realize the existence of a drop in acuity, ghost images, or general decrease in visual performance. A simple piece of tape over

the bifocal of the poorer eye can make a dramatic difference in visual and reading performance for the patient. Opaque or frosted tape, black electrical tape, lens frosting, increasing the bifocal power, and decreasing the bifocal power are all methods of aiding the suppression of the inhibiting eye. If the patient will not wear a patch, you may need to be creative to accomplish the goal of monocular reading, even considering the use of contact lenses. Some patients, especially those who have a better acuity in the nondominant eye, need to actually touch the eye to stop the inhibition. These people hold the lid of the poorer (previously dominant) eye closed with their fingers to see detail with their better eye. Sometimes this can be accomplished by stuffing tissue behind the lenses so there is a tactual sense to the occlusion process. This leaves the patient with both hands free and hopefully more comfortable while doing near tasks.

Visual Field Testing

Visual field testing with low vision patients is more of a functional test than a disease detection–oriented test. In most cases, the disease causing the vision loss is known and the fields are being taken to measure the extent of the impairment of visual functioning. Visual field testing will give you, the patient, and others an understanding of the field of view of the patient. You will use this information to determine the need to refer for orientation and mobility services (e.g., cane travel instruction). As with Amsler grid testing, you will look for severe constrictions that interfere with mobility; ring scotomas that interfere with near tasks, especially reading (these fields can simulate a severe field constriction even though far peripheral vision is evident); and peripheral islands of vision or location of scotomas that might interfere with device-assisted visual performance (e.g., right field loss, hemianopsias, multiple scotomas). For most patients with maculopathy, confrontation fields are an adequate assessment of the functional visual field. This condition does not typically affect the periphery, and thus a quick confirmation of an intact peripheral field is sufficient. The patient is seated 1 m from the clinician, normal room lighting is adequate, and a "count my fingers" target is more desirable than "see my wiggling fingers." (Refer to any text on visual fields for a full description of the test.)

Perimetry should be used with patients who show peripheral restrictions with confrontation testing. It should be noted that the clinician is not looking for subtle changes or losses of peripheral field. Large targets of 5–20 mm should be used to get a reliable response. (A III4e or equivalent target can be used as needed for documentation of legal blindness.) For patients with poor fixation, a cross can be used as a target to help maintain steady fixation during the test. The patient is instructed to look where the lines appear to cross. This also helps patients with nystagmus. Since this is a test of function, only eight to 12 meridians need to be tested. A simple arc perimeter with hand-held wand targets is an excellent instrument for this purpose (Figure 2.9). More sophisticated testing can be performed by modifying the targets and programs of some of the newer threshold visual field testing instrumentation.

A central threshold test can be successfully performed on a low vision patient. It provides invaluable information on the quality of central vision as well as the size and location of scotomas. This test maps the geography of the central retinal area in and around the PRL (Figure 2.10). This pictorial description of the viable retina may lead you to teach the patient strategies for eccentrically viewing. The PRL may be found to be encircled by scotomas or areas of depressed retina. Within the central 10 degrees, the PRL may be positioned to create a functional 1- or 2-degree central field. In this case, a different approach may be needed to find optimum performance at near. This functional field loss could be seen in the 20/60 patient that needs a closed-circuit television (CCTV) much like the patient with retinitis pigmentosa and a central field of a few degrees. The CCTV makes it easier to scan the material and to rapidly process visual information. If computerized or threshold tests are not available, a good tangent screen test can provide a wealth of information about the integrity of the visual fields, both centrally and peripherally. Do not wear the patient out trying to obtain extended information through visual field testing unless it is truly needed.

Visual Fields and the Low Vision Prescription

The evaluation of visual fields provides information regarding the extent of the intact central retina available for magnification and the extent of the loss of peripheral vision. Some conclusions follow:

- It is not helpful to magnify into areas of scotoma or within scotomas.
- Visual fields of 5 degrees or less may limit the amount of magnification from which a patient may benefit. The acuity will improve with 5× magnification, but the field of view is reduced functionally to 1 degree and the patient literally cannot find the object to be viewed through the system.
- Visual fields of 10 degrees or more do not usually limit magnification, although performance will be slower with higher levels.
- Mobility instruction should be considered when visual fields are reduced to below 40 degrees.

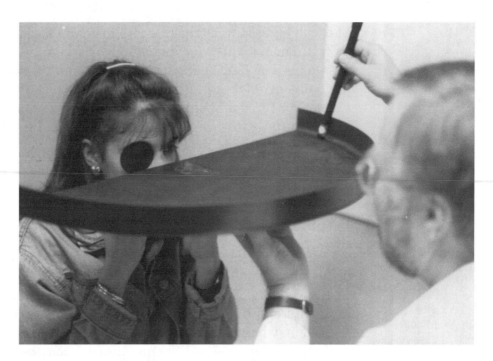

Figure 2.9. Perimetric testing is important to determine the presence of any functional field losses that may interfere with mobility or the use of prescribed devices. A simple way of measuring peripheral fields that will provide accurate functional information (as opposed to diagnostic testing) with a reasonable expenditure of time is shown here.

- Minification devices and peripheral field awareness systems should be considered when the visual fields are 5 degrees or less. If more field exists, it is often better to initiate scanning training. A gray area exists for successful use of these systems in patients with fields between 5 and 10 degrees. If the patient is very poor at scanning, the prisms or minifiers may provide some improved functioning. Remember, these systems are meant to make it easier for the patient to process visual information.
- Hemianopic losses will respond well to prisms and some of the newer mirror displacement systems.
- A patient who has 5-degree fields but retains some peripheral islands of vision is not a good candidate for prisms (perhaps minifiers). It is better to teach this patient to become aware of those peripheral islands of vision rather than to depend on prisms.
- Some states require 140 degrees of uninterrupted visual field to obtain a driver's license. For patients with macular degeneration, this may be available if the test is conducted with the patient eccentrically viewing the target (just above or below the scotoma).

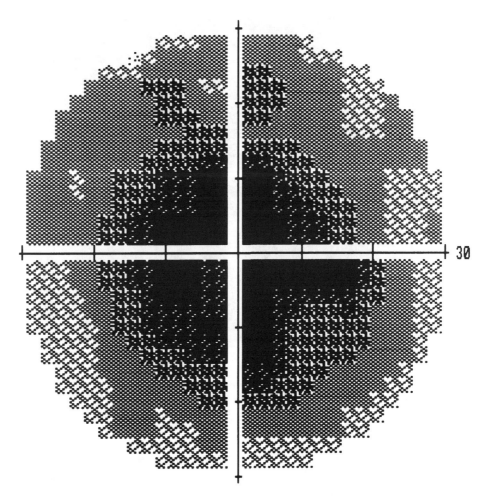

Figure 2.10. Automated threshold fields provide a much more detailed picture of the central area of functional vision. The test results in this figure indicate that the area most desirable for eccentric viewing is in the lower quadrant. Knowing this, the clinician can now guide the patient to an effective eccentric viewing position.

Color Vision Testing

Color vision testing is especially important for patients involved in vocational rehabilitation or in school. Here it is important to be aware of any color vision deficiencies. The easiest test is to have the patient match colors, as in the Holmgren wool test for color vision. A more scientific approach is the D-15 Dichotomous Test for color vision. Some patients respond well to the standard test chips, while others will provide more reliable responses when the large chip version of the test is used (Figure 2.11). Remember to note the lighting variables used. The chip test provides excellent functional data related to color vision problems that may affect the patient's ability to perform vocational and educational tasks and is easily administered. It is interpreted just as with the standard-size D-15 test. Some anecdotal successes have been reported with the use of various filters to improve the patient's awareness

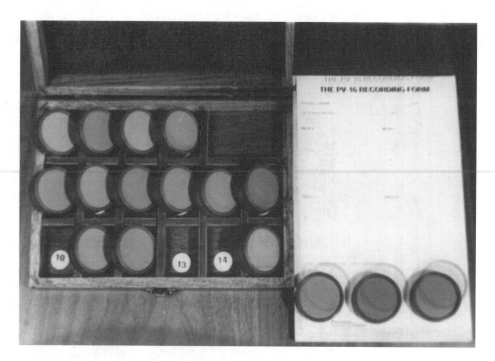

Figure 2.11. Even with large central scotomas and poor acuity, a patient will still exhibit some color vision or color-identifying capabilities. Using a color vision test like the one shown here from Precision Vision (Villa Park, IL) will identify serious functional problems in color vision that can interfere with a patient's vocational or educational goals.

of colors, but these are not practical treatment options. Color vision data is more often information for others and does not always impact on the actual treatment option. A color loss may prevent an individual from pursuing a driver's license or other vocational activities, however.

Ocular Health Testing

You are responsible for the ocular health of the patient as well as for the rehabilitative care; the two cannot be separated. The external evaluation is consistent with any other primary care testing—for example, eye movements, convergence near point, and pupil responses. These tests should be performed with the use of optical devices kept in mind. Extra time should be taken in describing the nystagmus and finding the null point (position of gaze where the nystagmus dampens) if one exists.

Many of these patients feel that because they have macular degeneration, they do not need to be concerned with checkups for glaucoma, cataracts, and so forth. You should perform tonometry and blood pressure measurements on patients, especially those who are not receiving ongoing eye care. The internal eye health examination should be performed at the end of the low vision examination because of light adaptation problems and the need for dilation. The exception would be when the history or initial data indicates the possibility of an active disease process in which there may be a need for referral for medical attention before initiating any rehabilitative care. The extent of the internal work-up depends on the information from the referring doctor and your confidence in that information, the date of the last examination, and the patient's report of vision changes. This testing is performed not to rediagnose, but simply to confirm those diseases that have been identified by the referring practitioner or to establish a reason for the visual impairment, if the patient is self-referred. Monocular direct and binocular indirect ophthalmoscopy with dilation are optimum tools for this procedure. (Remember, however, that just because you may not be able to see the retina does not mean the patient cannot see out. The media can often look much worse than the acuity reflects.)

Remember that the referring doctor follows the disease—you should concentrate on the vision rehabilitation aspects of the patient's care. The referring doctor should be included as one of the team members in the vision rehabilitation process. You should be careful when making statements about the disease, medical treatment, or surgical intervention. If you note something unusual, it is best to contact the referring doctor by phone or in writing with your questions. The additional data you receive from this communication will often clear up any concerns you have for the patient.

Other Tests

Occasionally, other testing is needed to provide a better measurement or description of the patient's impairment. The Brightness Acuity Test, ultrasound testing, electrodiagnostic testing, automated refraction, interferometry, and preferential looking testing are just a few of the additional tests that can provide more information about the patient. Any test that helps you better understand the functional implications of the patient's eye disease should be pursued.

PATIENT CONFERENCE

At this time, a demonstration of optical devices is in order, except in the following situations:

1. The patient needs eccentric viewing training. Proceed with this first and demonstrate the devices at the second visit, when a positive response is more probable.

2. A simple bifocal add increase is being prescribed.
3. A patch is needed for one bifocal to eliminate retinal rivalry.

The data collected should be explained to the patient because most are curious about why a whole examination was performed instead of just looking at magnifiers. Let the patient know that you will prescribe a system that is unique. As part of the diagnostic procedure you are testing responses to selected optical systems. Based on the data collected and the responses, you will prescribe a device that addresses the primary goal. Both of you then have an opportunity to work with these special lenses and systems in a more natural setting to determine whether they will be effective and practical for the patient. You should reinforce to the patient that you do not want to prescribe a pair of glasses or a low vision device(s) that will end up sitting on a bureau. This assures the patient that you are taking the extra time to make sure the devices will be used. Most important, you make the patient a full partner in the decision-making process. Having done this, you are ready to start the low vision device evaluation.

Low Vision Device Evaluation
Once you have completed the low vision examination, you should be ready to test your patient's ability to use various low vision devices. The evaluation is based on the patient's particular goals. Thus, either distance or near low vision devices should be evaluated. Ultimately, both distance and near vision might be evaluated, but the patient's primary goal should be addressed first. Remember, not all individuals will be able to attain their goals. Keep in mind the availability of other rehabilitative sources as well as other nonvisual means of communication (e.g., books on tape, radio).

You should start with the magnification derived from either the distance acuity, near acuity, or a combination of both, and modify that based on Amsler grid testing, contrast sensitivity data, lighting conditions, and any other factor that you think might make a difference in success.

The sequence you develop will be personal. The following is an overview of magnification assessment. Remember to move toward the patient's goal.

Distance Low Vision Device Evaluation
Patients with 20/100 acuity or better should be given a 2.5× monocular telescope. A patient's acuity is expected to improve 2.5 times with this telescope (i.e., 20/100 VA should increase to approximately 20/40). Patients with VAs between 20/100 and 20/300 should be tested with a 4× or a 6× unit, and those with VAs from 20/300 to 20/600 should use an 8× unit. Persons with acuities

worse than 20/600 should not be considered for telescopes, at least for the initial prescription. They may be candidates for binoculars or special training.

VA	Telescope
≤20/100	2.5×
20/120–20/300	4–6×
20/300–20/600	8–10×
≥20/600	—

To help your patients with distance viewing, focus the telescope on the test chart first and then present it to the patient. Have the patient use the telescope to find you standing next to the chart and then follow your hand to the chart. This will reduce the patient's initial frustration in trying to locate a small chart in a big room through the small field afforded by the telescope. (Note: Nystagmus is not a contraindication to successful use of telescopes. A white ring painted on the ocular housing will improve fixation.) The best responses are indicated when the patient obtains the appropriate increase in acuity and has minimal difficulty in locating objects through the device. Patients who obtain the correct improvement in acuity but cannot localize or focus with the device may need long-term training. Telescopes can easily be dispensed and loaned (with appropriate training) to the patient who demonstrates an ability to use the unit in this initial evaluation.

Using the telescope in this diagnostic sequence will provide information about the response of the patient to telescopic magnification, the use of the telescope, and the potential for using a telescope to solve the patient's specific problems.

Near Low Vision Device Evaluation

As indicated earlier, evaluation of the initial near point acuities can be performed with the Lighthouse Near Acuity Chart. There are also other charts to do this. You will eventually settle on a chart with which you are comfortable. For this discussion, we use the Lighthouse Chart. This chart records acuities in M notation and is designed to aid you in selecting the appropriate level of magnification. It has large, isolated letters that promote success for the initial measurement.

The patient should hold the card at 40 cm and read the smallest line possible. For the initial diagnostic sequence, the endpoint acuity of 1 M (20/50) is arbitrarily selected. Because M notations are linear, if the patient reads 5 M print and the ability to read 1 M print is desired, 5× magnification is required. The print is moved to ⅕ distance (i.e., 40/5 = 8 cm) to obtain this magnification. A +12.50 D lens is needed to provide a clear image at this distance (available accommodation may allow a weaker spectacle lens in the final prescription). This lens represents 5× magnification. To simplify the process, the right side of the chart indicates the dioptric power of the lens needed to provide 1 M acuity. Thus, at the right margin of the chart for the patient reading at an acuity of 5 M at 40 cm, the notation is +12.00 D. This is the add that should be placed in the trial frame. The patient is instructed to read the chart at the appropriate 8.5-cm working distance. (The card should be presented at 8.5 cm, and the patient moves it in and out slowly to obtain better focus.) Deviations from the appropriate working distance may be indicative of uncorrected distant refractive errors, accommodation, and so forth. For instance, if the patient reports clear vision at 6 cm instead of 8 cm, a possibility of 4.50 D of uncorrected myopia is indicated. The 6-cm distance indicates a demand of 16.60 D (100/6 = 16.60 D) instead of 12.00 D. The difference could be 4.60 D of uncorrected myopia or the patient accommodating 4.60 D to obtain more magnification.

If the patient cannot respond to any letters at 40 cm, hold the chart at 20 cm and use twice the indicated dioptric value from your microscopic trial lens. The use of your trial lenses and a microscopic trial kit (Volk, Designs for Vision, Keeler, etc.) will allow you to demonstrate microscopic magnification from +4.00 D to +100.00 D.

A demonstration of improved acuity should be accomplished with almost every patient you treat. Additionally, to help others understand the functional use of the magnifier you should refer to the Freeman Functional Near Field Chart (Westbury Consulting, Pittsburgh, PA). This clearly demonstrates the small field of view that accompanies the improvement in acuity (see Form 2.3).

Once the level of magnification is determined with the Lighthouse Chart, a second acuity measurement of reading ability should be taken. A patient who can see 1 M single letters may or may not be able to read paragraph material of equivalent size. There are many reading cards available. Use the one you are comfortable with and hold it at the same working distance as you did the Lighthouse Chart. The authors have found that the Hoeft near chart (Wayne Hoeft, Los Angeles, CA) provides valuable information as well as encouragement to the patient.

Begin with a paragraph twice as large as the letters read successfully on the Lighthouse Chart. Poor performance on the reading card may indicate the following:

1. A need for more magnification
2. A need for eccentric viewing training

3. A resistance to the close working distance
4. An academic problem with the reading task

If the patient is having difficulty reading the sentences, try using a typoscope. If the patient's responses improve, the problem area is most likely one of contrast or eccentric viewing. Increased magnification, in this case, will improve acuity but will not resolve the underlying problem or improve visual performance. The patient will be happy with the demonstration's success, but you will need to achieve this success for the patient with a prescriptive program of contrast enhancement and/or eccentric viewing training.

Sometimes you will not want to use 1 M as the target. The patient may have a specific reading task in mind, and your success will be greater if that particular print size can be read. Table 2.1 provides a comparison between acuities and actual material that can be seen with that level of acuity. This will be a tremendous help to you in obtaining this very important positive first response.

Filter Evaluation

The evaluation of filter systems must be individual. The patient may be able to give you a feel for what is comfortable in the office and even outside during your initial evaluation but, for a true evaluation, the patient should be allowed to borrow the filters for a few days. This allows patients to experience the filters in their day-to-day environment. When the patient returns, you will know whether the filters are appropriate or need to be darker, lighter, or a different shade. NOIR (South Lyon, MI) and Corning (Corning, NY) are the most commonly used filters for evaluation. Remember to consider the factors of glare control, light transmission, and wavelength (color) when selecting a specific filter.

Instructions on the proper use of sun filters will be invaluable to the patient. Specifically, the patient should put on the filter as the threshold leading to the outside is crossed. This maintains a reasonably constant level of light, requiring less light adaptation time. Conversely, when a patient enters a building, the sun filters should be removed just as the patient crosses the threshold. When using filters this way, patients note definite improvements in ease when traveling between indoors and outdoors.

First Visit Conclusion

At the completion of the initial evaluation encourage the patient to think about what has transpired during the evaluation. A summary of the evaluation and findings are given. You should have reviewed the optical and nonoptical options which introduced the patient to immediate VA success. Now the real work begins. Success as defined by your optics is only marginally valuable to the success

Table 2.1. Table of Approximate Equivalent Visual Acuity Notations for Near[a]

Meters equivalent	Snellen equivalent	Jaeger[b]	AMA notation	Lower-case point	Approx. height (in mm)	Visual angle (in min)	Usual type text size[c]	Equivalent reading acuity[d]
0.4 M	20/20	—	14/14	3	0.58	5	—	—
0.5 M	20/25	J1–J2	14/17.5	4	0.75	6.25	Footnotes	Paperback/newsprint
0.8 M	20/40	J4–J5	14/28	6	1.15	10	Paperback print	Magazines
1.0 M	20/50	J6	14/35	8	1.5	12.5	Newspaper print	High school texts
1.2 M	20/60	J8	14/42	10	1.75	15	Magazine print	Children's books
1.6 M	20/80	J9–J11	14/56	14	2.3	20	Children's books	Large-print materials
2.0 M	20/100	J11–J12	14/70	18	3	25	Large-print material	—
4.0 M	20/200	J17	14/140	36	6	50	Newspaper subheadlines	—
5.0 M	20/250	J18	14/175	—	7.5	62.5	Newspaper headlines	—
10.0 M	20/500	J19	14/350	—	15	124	0.5-in. letter	—
20.0 M	20/1,000	—	14/700	—	30	250	1-in. letter	—

[a]There will be differences in the numbers presented in various published charts. This is indicative of the lack of standardization in charts and varying clinical experiences. (R Jose, R Atcherson. Standardization of near point acuity cards. Am J Optom Physiol Optic 1977;54:540.)

[b]There can be as much as a 25% difference in size of letters, works, etc. from one Jaeger chart to another.

[c]This refers to the comparison of letter size. Indicates vision needed for reading labels and other short-term identification tasks.

[d]This refers to the acuity needed in order for most patients to comfortably read the indicated materials. Calculations based on review of clinical charts at University of Houston.

Source: Dr. Richard Brilliant, Wm. Feinbloom Vision Rehabilitation Center, and Dr. Randall Jose, University of Houston, College of Optometry.

that the patient must experience in the real world. The patient now has to incorporate the information you have given and the optical and nonoptical success that you have demonstrated into his or her ADL. A recommendation for the patient to return for continued evaluation and design of a training protocol including the use of loaner equipment should be discussed and encouraged.

The additional visits, which typically last 30–60 minutes, can be thought of as psychophysically monitoring the ocular disease. You, and now the patient, have the use of sophisticated optical and nonoptical systems—including, but not limited to, microscopes, telescopes, hand magnifiers, stand magnifiers, electro-optical systems, lighting, and field enhancers—to help the patient functionally and to help you medically follow the disease by noting any change in responses. With these systems, the patient's perception of changes in the pathology, real or imagined, can be monitored. Any changes should be reported to the patient's primary care eye doctor for further evaluation and management as well as to the patient's primary care general practitioner for any systemic evaluation. Sometimes these reviews also lead to suggestions of counseling for help in adjusting to the difficulties the patient is experiencing.

At this stage, your initial report should be sent to the referring doctor. Forwarding reports to the doctor keeps communication open. It can also lead to interesting information about the patient's relationship with the referring or attending doctor. Patients who do not want a letter forwarded may tell you that they have not told the doctor that they were coming to your office or may feel unsure of the doctor's response because the doctor told them nothing more could be done. If the patient arrived thinking that low vision services are not in the mainstream of ophthalmic care because of comments from the primary care doctor, it can make prescribing more challenging and your goals for the patient more difficult to accomplish.

FORM DESCRIPTIONS

2.1 Examination Form

The examination form is used to help you gather information during the visit. It contains the compiled results found throughout your initial examination. This data will lead you through the history and those tests necessary to establish a base for working with optical and nonoptical treatment options. At the conclusion of the examination period, the patient's prognosis for success will be established and treatment options discussed. Both private practice (Form 2.1a) and clinical setting (Form 2.1b) formats are included.

2.2 Jose Eccentric Viewing Home Training Kit

The Jose Eccentric Viewing Home Training Kit (Spalding Magnifiers and Mattingly International) was designed to enhance eccentric viewing capability expeditiously. It can be used by the patient both in the office and at home. Successful completion of this process should result in enhanced performance with low vision device prescriptions.

The ability of the patient to view eccentrically is very important to the determination of a proper treatment option. If the patient is diagnosed as having poor or nonexistent eccentric viewing skills, a home training program can be dispensed that will help the patient develop these skills as well as become comfortable with a closer work distance and learn to read with magnification and a smaller field of view. This kit has been designed by one of the authors (RTJ) and consists of a clip board, training materials, and stand magnifier (see Figure 2.7). The random letter sheet from the training exercises in the training section of this book is used with the kit. An additional page with short words is added along with a third page that includes two columns of words and engages the patient in some saccadic eye movements as he or she finds the word in column 1 and moves to column 2 to find another word. The patient is instructed to set a timer for 15 minutes and to not work any longer. The patient is to perform the task three times per day. If the patient wishes to perform more exercises, it is better to do more 15-minute sessions than three longer sessions. The text size used depends on the acuity and patient difficulty reading the letters. The kit comes with a 5× or a 7× stand magnifier. It is preferable to use the higher-power stand magnifier and smaller print. This forces the patient to a more exacting fixation to perform the exercises. Although a misnomer, the patient is told that these exercises are "muscle" exercises, so it won't be confused with a reading or acuity exercise or even a treatment option. This is very important because some of the patients will be able to see the letters with their bifocal correction or low-power magnifier and do not understand the purpose of the training; they may feel that you "sold" them a useless kit.

The task is for the patient to find the first letter at the beginning of the first line and move the magnifier across the line, identifying each letter as he or she goes along. At first, most patients cannot finish more than 10–12 lines in the 15-minute period. They are given 2–3 weeks of home training and told that they are expected only to complete the first page. They are always to do the first page or letter page and, if they finish the page, they can repeat it from the top or try to identify words on the second page. The real eccentric viewing training comes when identifying the letters. The exercise is described as "push-ups" for the eye muscles, so they can find the right spot on the retina for best vision and learn how to hold that spot (so the vision will not flash on and off, as so many report). Like push-ups, these are very simple but effective exercises, if done faithfully. They can also be very boring, so the other pages are added to break up the monotony. Also, advise the caretaker and the patient's family member that the patient does not need to call out each letter correctly for the exercise to be effective. Remember, this is a muscle exercise, not a vision exercise. Otherwise, these helpers will stand over the patient creating anxiety for both coach and patient. Almost all patients will come back in 2 weeks with improved eccentric viewing skills, improved attitude about the prognosis for their vision, and less resistance to a close work distance (most start holding the magnifier closer so that more can be seen and the exercises can be finished more quickly). Most patients will now be able to do some reading (the single-letter and paragraph acuities are more equal). At the second visit, you can proceed with the prescription of a microscope or telescope with better response and a much higher probability of success. The biggest problem you will have with this exercise protocol is that, because it is so simple, many patients do not believe it will work and do not comply. Sending them back for a second 2 weeks and a stern warning to "do it right this time" can be very effective.

2.3 Freeman Functional Near Field Chart

The Freeman Functional Near Field Chart is designed to determine the functional size of the usable field of a near magnifier (i.e., handheld, stand, telemicroscopic, head-borne, or electronic). The extent of the field can be demonstrated to the patient and others without having the patient read a word or grasp a concept. The card can also be used to measure vertical fields.

This chart is not meant to plot out degrees of scotoma, nor is the spacing between the numbers and letters meant to determine distance between printed letters. These charts were developed clinically, and the distance between numbers and letters is meant only to decrease confusion due to the crowding phenomenon. All diagnostic information should be collected before this measurement.

This information is useful in the following situations:

1. At the conclusion of a near evaluation with low vision devices
2. As a teaching and training technique before prescribing a near prescription
3. As a method to monitor changes of near usable field

Instructions for Use of the Card

1. Place the card parallel to the near low vision device and the patient's face. Make sure the card is at the focal length of the lens. If used with a stand magnifier or CCTV, interpose a reading or bifocal correction (when necessary) to compensate for diverging light from the stand magnifier or CCTV.
2. Position the lighting to achieve best illumination for use of the device.
3. With the patient viewing the center dot or where the center dot would appear to be, ask him or her to tell you the farthest number and letter that can be seen clearly to either side. If there is a central or paracentral scotoma, have the patient use an eccentric position to see the central area. This might produce a lopsided field but will be of value for patient awareness when performing other near tasks. This card can be used to teach eccentric viewing using conventional eccentric viewing techniques as well.
4. Measure this distance linearly on the chart. For example, C,3; B,4; and so forth.
5. Place a word or words in that space. The size of the letter or words should be based on the metric near point findings from the low vision evaluation. An alternative to placing a word in the space is to take this finding and demonstrate it in a newspaper or magazine. This will show the patient and others this measurement in the context of printed material. It will also show the patient how difficult hyphenated words, lengthy words, or unfamiliar words will be. It is most important to remember that seeing print size and determining a usable field is not synonymous with reading.
6. Repeat the test vertically.

Summary

By using this card you will demonstrate linear dimensions of both the horizontal and vertical usable field of the low vision device being recommended. Changing lighting, posture, vertex distance, and other variables and remeasuring the near field will help the patient understand the importance of maintaining correct focal distances. The more the patient understands the functional-optical properties of the device, the more proficient he or she will become in using it.

2.4 Follow-Up Letter

A letter must be sent to the referring physician for two reasons: (1) It helps the doctor know what has been done and how successful you were (prognosis for the patient), and (2) it is good public relations—keeping the referral process intact. You will eventually want to draft your own letters, but the two examples provided here will steer you in the right direction.

REFERENCES

1. Shindell S, Clinical Psychologist, Western Blind Rehabilitation Center, Palo Alto Veterans Administration Medical Center, Palo Alto, CA. Handout on Communication Skills.
2. Freeman P, Jose R. Diagnostic patching for the profoundly multiply handicapped, visually impaired child (PMHVI). J Behav Optom 1995;6(9):59.

SUGGESTED READING

Cole R, Rosenthal B. Remediation and Management of Low Vision. St. Louis: Mosby, 1996.

Faye E. Clinical Low Vision. Boston: Little, Brown, 1984.

Goodrich G, Jose RT, Ariditi A. Low Vision—The Reference. New York: The Lighthouse, 1996.

Gottlieb D, Allen C, Eikenberry J, et al. Living with Vision Loss. Atlanta: St. Barthalemy Press, 1996.

Jose RT. Understanding Low Vision. New York: American Foundation for the Blind, 1982.

Jose RT (ed). Journal of Vision Rehabilitation. Kansas City: Torozzolo Publications.

The Journal of Visual Impairment and Blindness. New York: American Foundation for the Blind.

Kirschner C. Data on Blindness and Visual Impairment in the United States. New York: American Foundation for the Blind, 1985.

Mehr E, Freid A. Low Vision Care. Chicago: Professional, 1975.

Newsletter of the Low Vision Section of the American Optometric Association.

Nowakowski R. Primary Low Vision Care. East Norwalk, CT: Appleton & Lange, 1994.

Rosenthal B, Cole R. Functional Assessment of Low Vision. St. Louis: Mosby, 1996.

Formal History Summary

Patient name: _____ Date: _____

Chief complaint:

Visual history/medical history/family history/social history:

Allergies (medicines, eye drops, etc.):

Concerns about mobility/distance vision:

Depth perception: Difficulties?   Y   N   Explain:

Concerns about near vision:

Illumination:

Work/hobbies:

Primary goal:

Secondary goal:

Medical History

1.   When was your last physical? _____ Doctor: _____
2.   How did the doctor say your health was?
3.   What is your opinion of your health?
4.   Do you have any allergies? If so, please list.

Do you or any members of your family have problems with the following (S = self, F = family)?

1.   Heart: S   F
     a. How long?
     b. Medications: _____

2.   Circulation: S   F
     a. How long?
     b. Medications: _____

3.   Kidneys: S   F
     a. How long?
     b. Medications: _____

4.   Liver: S   F
     a. How long?
     b. Medications: _____

5.   Lungs: S   F
     a. How long?
     b. Medications: _____

6.   Skin conditions: S   F
     a. How long?
     b. Medications: _____

7.   Hypertension: S   F
     a. How long?
     b. Medications: _____

8.   Neurologic disease: S   F
     a. How long?
     b. Medications: _____

9.   Endocrine: S   F
     a. How long?
     b. Medications: _____

10. Diabetes: S   F
     a. How long have you been diabetic?
     b. How is your diabetes controlled?
        1) Diet
        2) Oral medication
        3) Insulin   What type?   Dosage?
     c. How is your glucose monitored?
        1) Urine strip   Average reading: _____

    2) Glucometer   Average reading: _____
    3) A$_1$C (glycosylated hemoglobin)
    4) Physician   How often? _____
  d. How often do you become hypo/hyperglycemic?
  e. Are you a member of the American Diabetes Association?

11. Gastrointestinal: S   F
  a. How long?
  b. Medications: _____

12. Musculoskeletal: S   F
  a. How long?
  b. Medications: _____

13. Stroke: S   F
  a. How long?
  b. Medications: _____

14. Depression: S   F
  a. How long?
  b. Medications: _____

15. Traumatic head injury: S   F
  a. How long?
  b. Medications: _____

16. Other: S   F
  a. How long?
  b. Medications: _____

Visual History
1. How long ago did you first know you had a vision problem?
2. When was your last eye examination?
3. Who was your doctor?
4. Were your eyes dilated?
5. Have you ever had treatment or surgery for your eyes?
6. Are you taking eye medications?
7. Have you had recent changes in your vision?
8. Have you ever had a low vision evaluation?
9. Who was your doctor?
10. What have your doctors told you was the cause of your vision problem? Explain your problem.
11. Do you wear glasses now? If so, do they help?
12. How well do you think you see now?
13. Is there any family history of glaucoma, cataract, blindness, or any other eye problem?

Psychosocial History
1. What is your present living situation?
2. Are you able to take care of yourself?
3. What was the last school grade you completed?
4. Do you smoke now?   Y   N
   a. If yes, how much?
   b. Have you smoked for 1 year or more?   Y   N
5. Have you had any rehabilitation training? Do you use assistive devices?
6. What social or recreational programs are you involved in?
7. Who helps with your transportation?
8. Where do you get support? (family, friends, etc.)
9. How do you feel about your vision loss?

Mobility History
1. Can you see well enough to get around outdoors?
2. Do you drive?
3. Do you have mobility aids—for example, a cane or a guide dog?
4. Do you have glasses or optical devices that help you get around?
5. Do you have difficulty getting around indoors?
6. Do you tend to trip over low objects, such as curbs or steps?
7. Do you tend to bump into objects at eye level?
8. Do you bump one side of your body more than the other?

Distance Vision History

	At what distance?	With what device?
1. Are you able to see		
a. Billboards?	_____	_____
b. Labels?	_____	_____
c. Faces?	_____	_____
2. Do you attend movies?	_____	_____
3. Do you watch TV?	_____	_____
What is the screen size?	_____	_____
4. Do you have problems recognizing colors? If so, please explain.		

Activities of Daily Living
Because of your vision loss, do you have difficulty
- Doing your housework?
- Seeing to cook?
- Seeing stove dials?
- Seeing the flame on the stove?
- Seeing food on your plate?
- Seeing the number pad on the telephone?
- Seeing to groom yourself?

Near Vision History

	At what distance?	With what device?
1. Do you read print?		
2. Can you read		
a. Newspaper headlines?	_____	_____
b. Large print?	_____	_____
c. Textbooks?	_____	_____
d. Typeset print?	_____	_____
e. Magazines?	_____	_____
f. Newspapers?	_____	_____
g. Telephone book?	_____	_____

3. How much reading do you do now?
4. Which size print do you use most?
5. What kind of light do you use for reading?
6. Did you read more before your vision loss?
7. Do you want to read more than you presently do?

Illumination
1. Do you see better and are your eyes more comfortable when it is bright and sunny or overcast and cloudy?
2. Do you wear sunglasses?
3. Do you use a visor (hat)?
4. Are you bothered by glare?
5. Do you have more trouble with your vision at night than during the day?
6. Do you use extra light to improve your vision?

Work, School, and Hobbies
1. Are you involved in any of the following activities now or were you before your vision loss?
   a. Sewing
   b. Crocheting
   c. Playing cards
   d. Playing a musical instrument
   e. Swimming
   f. Bowling
   g. Bicycling
   h. Typing—computers
   i. Minor repairs
   j. Other
2. Do you have any particular difficulties at school or work because of your vision?
3. Do you have any particular difficulties around the house because of your vision?
4. How do you spend your day?
5. What are some of your major activities?
6. If your vision can be improved with optical devices, are there special tasks that you would like to be able to do?

S/F* VAs w/wo Lighting PH
OD _____ / _____ / _____
OS _____ / _____ / _____
OU _____ / _____ / _____

Metric VAs w/wo Lighting Dist.
OD _____ / _____ / _____
OS _____ / _____ / _____
OU _____ / _____ / _____

Rx
OD _____
OS _____
Add _____

Amsler Grid screening _____
OD _____ OS _____ OU _____

Mobility screening _____ Light _____
OD _____ OS _____ OU _____
2 quadrants   2 quadrants   2 quadrants
4 quadrants   4 quadrants   4 quadrants
simultaneous   simultaneous   simultaneous
counting fingers   counting fingers   counting fingers

External evaluation: OD S/F/J   OS S/F/J   PERRLA   CNP _____   Suppression/Diplopia R/G
Cover test: Distance _____ Near _____
Other:

Lighting _____
Refraction A/R   Subjective   VAs   Add   VAs   Distance
OD _____ _____ / _____ / _____ / _____ / _____
OS _____ _____ / _____ / _____ / _____ / _____

Slit Lamp

Anterior segment OD	Anterior segment OS
Eyelids	Eyelids
Lacrimal gland	Lacrimal gland
Cornea	Cornea
Iris	Iris
Orbit	Orbit
Lens	Lens
Anterior chamber	Anterior chamber
Post segment	Post segment
Media (vitreous)	Media (vitreous)
Macula	Macula
Disc	Disc
Blood vessels	Blood vessels
Periphery	Periphery

Tonometry: OD _____ OS _____

Internal Evaluation:
Dilated/Undilated   Direct +20, +60, +90   Time _____ Agent_____

OD   OS

Other Tests:
PAM   TAG   FFNF   Glare   Gonioscopy   Scleral depression   Fields   Color screening
D-15   Binocular testing   Worth four-dot   Stereo—gross/fine   Electro testing   CSF testing
Keratometry   Other
Results:

*Snellen/Feinbloom.

Form 2.1a *(continued)*

Low Vision Devices

OD	OS

Distance

Near

Filters

Electro-optical

Counsel and education time: _____

Plan:

A.   Discussion of medical condition:

_____ Prognosis
_____ Alternative medical options (e.g., surgery, laser, medical prescription, nonmedical prescription)
_____ Review of test results—distance and near visual acuities—nature of disease

B.   Functional visual concerns:

_____ OK to use eyes (they cannot be worn out)
_____ Close television viewing will not hurt eyes

_____ Fear of total blindness unfounded
_____ Driving—visually legal/visually illegal
_____ Not able to have conventional Rx

C.   Optical/nonoptical options:

_____ Importance of practice in acquiring adaptive skills
_____ Lighting
_____ Contrast
_____ Working distance
_____ Eccentric viewing
_____ Principles of magnification
     RSM   RDM
_____ Specific reading techniques
_____ Electronic devices
_____ Specific ADL adaptations

D.   Psychological/social factors:

_____ Independence
_____ Importance of acuity
_____ Emotional reaction
_____ Attitude
_____ Ability to deal with the challenge

E.   Contact doctor: _____ (Contact this doctor first, then contact us if any problems occur.)

F.   Recommended devices for the patient:

Schedule with doctor/assistant   Date: _____
Noncovered Y/N $ _____   Fee Y/N $ _____

                                        _____
                                        Signature

Consultation/New Visit

Patient name: _____ Attend. intern: _____

Accompanied by: _____ Assist. intern: _____

Date: _____

Record Review	Medical/Health History	Patient History
	Last medical examination	
	Doctor	
	General health	
	Heart/blood pressure	
	Metabolic/diabetes	
	Arthritis	
	Neurologic	
	Hearing/other sensory	
	Stroke	
	Respiratory	
	Immune system	
	Tumors	
	Injuries/physical disabilities	

Visual History

Last eye examination

Next appt. scheduled

Doctor/clinic

Diagnosis

Onset

Medical/surgical treatment

Previous spectacle Rx

Previous low vision Rx

Family history

Changes in vision

Ocular Side Effects (PDR)	Medications	Condition	Dose
	_____	_____	_____
	_____	_____	_____
	_____	_____	_____
	_____	_____	_____
	_____	_____	_____

Psychosocial History (address past and present for all concerns)
Living situation
Rehabilitation training
Other assistive devices
Active in social recreational activities (church)
Patient attitude toward vision loss
Family support
Financial problems
Transportation (who helps)

Task Analysis
Circle one for each: Y = yes, problematic; N = no problem; S = somewhat problematic

Traveling: Do you have difficulty

Traveling locally alone?	Y	N	S
Traveling far alone?	Y	N	S
Seeing to drive a car?	Y	N	S
Seeing traffic lights?	Y	N	S
Seeing street signs?	Y	N	S
Crossing streets?	Y	N	S

Distance viewing: Do you have difficulty

Getting around people?	Y	N	S
Getting around objects?	Y	N	S
Seeing curbs and stairs?	Y	N	S
Walking without falling?	Y	N	S
Seeing faces?	Y	N	S
Seeing the television?	Y	N	S
Seeing live theater?	Y	N	S

ADL: Do you have difficulty

Doing housework?	Y	N	S
Cooking?	Y	N	S
Seeing stove dials?	Y	N	S
Seeing stove flame?	Y	N	S
Seeing food on your plate?	Y	N	S
Seeing the phone dial?	Y	N	S
Seeing to groom yourself?	Y	N	S

Near tasks: Do you have difficulty

Reading headlines?	Y	N	S
Reading large print?	Y	N	S
Reading books?	Y	N	S
Reading newsprint?	Y	N	S
Seeing prices and labels?	Y	N	S
Reading your mail?	Y	N	S
Signing your name/checks?	Y	N	S
Seeing colors?	Y	N	S
Filling a syringe (diabetic)?	Y	N	S
Seeing medical labels?	Y	N	S
Seeing to sew/knit/crochet?	Y	N	S
Seeing to play cards/bingo?	Y	N	S
With household repairs?	Y	N	S

Lighting: Do you have difficulty

Tolerating the sun?	Y	N	S
On cloudy/rainy days?	Y	N	S
In dim light?	Y	N	S

Do you wear sunglasses?	Y	N	S
Are they effective?	Y	N	S
Does bright light help you?	Y	N	S

Preferred light sources: (circle)

Incandescent   Fluorescent   Halogen

Form 2.1b *(continued)*

Consultation/New Visit
Unaided VA

OD _____ OS _____ OU _____   Chart:

Distance Rx   VA   Chart (   )   PD (   )   SV   BIF   TRI

OD _____

OS _____

Binocularity: **External:** (pupils, EOM, null)

Confrontation field: Perimetry _____

LV Refraction: **P.H.** _____
Retinoscopy:
Subjective:
New VA: OD _____ OS _____ OU _____ No change ____ Telescope _____
CSF screening:
Better eye (OD, OS):
Binocular: _____

	Near Acuity	Bifocal/Rx	Single letter:	Paragraph:
OD (SC) (CC)				
OS (SC) (CC)				
OU (SC) (CC)				

Amsler   **OD**   **Amsler**   **OS**

Test distance: _____   Test distance: _____

Color screening: D-15   **Near CSF:**

Other devices/options:
1)   3)
2)   4)

Morbidity/Functional Priorities

1. _____   3. _____

2. _____   4. _____

Near Assessment   (OD OS OU)   Field of view   _____ M

```
                    5
                    4
                    3
                    2
                    1
  9 8 7 6 5 4 3 2 1 X A B C D E F G H
                    A
                    B
                    C
                    D
                    E
```

Tentative Rx: _____

VA: _____   (single letter, paragraph)

Reading performance: _____

_____

_____

Intermediate Assessment   (OD OS OU)   Field of view   _____ M

```
                    5
                    4
                    3
                    2
                    1
  9 8 7 6 5 4 3 2 1 X A B C D E F G H
                    A
                    B
                    C
                    D
                    E
```

Tentative Rx:

VA: _____   (single letter, paragraph)

Distance Assessment   (OD OS OU)

Tentative Rx: Eye _____   VA _____   FOV _____

Form 2.1b *(continued)*

Lighting/Contrast Assessment

OD   OS

Fundus   Slit Lamp

Primary Dx: Secondary Dx: IOP:_____ Time:_____ Drug:_____
OD:_____   OD:_____   OD:_____
OS:_____   OS:_____   OS:_____

Prognosis: [ ] excellent   [ ] good   [ ] guarded   [ ] poor

Summary/Goals

Plan Next Visit

Special Tests				**Patient Management Actions**		
					Need	Completed
Perimetry	[ ]	DFE	[ ]	Med referral	[ ]	[ ]
C10-2	[ ]	Photo	[ ]	OD referral	[ ]	[ ]
C24-2	[ ]	ADL	[ ]	Soc. work referral	[ ]	[ ]
Glare	[ ]	Research candidate	[ ]	Educ. referral	[ ]	[ ]
CSF	[ ]	BAT	[ ]	Multicare referral	[ ]	[ ]
				Tech. ctr. referral	[ ]	[ ]
				Rehab. referral	[ ]	[ ]
				CCTV-demo	[ ]	[ ]
				Mentor needed	[ ]	[ ]
				Mentor candidate	[ ]	[ ]
				Psych. referral	[ ]	[ ]
				Other referral	[ ]	[ ]

Attending clinician: _____   Date: _____   Next visit: _____

Eccentric Viewing Training Materials

You are about to practice a new way of using your vision. It may be difficult at first, but persistence is also a key to success.

This kit includes the following:

1. Stand magnifier
2. Printed materials of varying difficulty

INSTRUCTIONS

1. Place the printed material on a flat, even surface. The clipboard provided is ideal.
2. Place the stand magnifier flat on the page. This is the optimal position for proper focusing.
3. Move the magnifier and printed material to a distance that allows you to see the print.
4. Be sure to have a bright light directed down onto the material. Illumination is *essential* to the success of the program.
5. The text gradually becomes more difficult. As you master each page, continue on to the next.
6. Practice for 15 minutes at a time. If you tire, take frequent breaks. Do this three times per day for no longer than 15 minutes each time.

If you have any questions, do not hesitate to contact us.

Low Vision Reading Exercise (8 Point)

K Q U O G C A H F P B V T D L Z X J I M S Y W N R H W S M

G S B D L X R J F C I W O N Q P T D Z V E H A G U K B Q P

W J E X Q I Z G C M S U F B H Y A V D L K N T P R O H Y I

N Y V E A R I M X G O U D H T Z K Q S W B J L F C P D O P

Q O C X F L A B E Y A W J T P N Z K M D T S V U G E R N I

A F H P B S E X F T R Q N Z M J I L M S T D L O R Z T P L E

T L D X Z J M S W N T Y R F H R P B V L E Z I U P B M N R T

a j f z h x r d a l p t b v q n k y u w s o y g m c l m s t z h l c m

c w s o m z n d t q v p b e h x l a r g i g j i r k m n p o q r t w

s p c b l e x f r g o q y n v z w k m u j i t a d h d s g l k e t y l

b s l x r f c w o n q p t d m z s y k g u a e h v k q u d p l m o n

v d t k x n v b r w i t o p w q c r u g r n l p q r s t w v y u o x n

f p u o h g d x z m e t l q r k a w e s w r c f p o z i r c r w r g l

1 9 0 2 3 4 8 5 4 7 5 8 9 1 4 3 7 6 9 4 8 3 2 5 9 7 5 6 7 2 3 4 6

1 5 u y 8 u 0 e 4 5 x 6 v 7 b 8 n 9 m 0 1 s 2 d 3 f 4 g 5 h 6 g 7 j

v d t k m z i p n j w a y h n h b r e f l x c q g u s l g i p r q w m

f p u o h g d x z m t l q r k w a s e v j n b y l f c p o z t r p u m

1 c 8 x 2 9 v 5 i b 3 r 5 o 7 p b 4 5 i v 9 j 6 m 4 r s 6 y p 3 c q

f t b p h k y n a l v d z q i x g j m e c w u r s o c k l r u b v r t y

a j f z h x r d a l w y n y r h k q u o g c a f h r p e b v z d r s l t

i 8 0 3 5 j o 8 6 j 4 p e 3 2 0 j 8 h 9 x 4 2 c v b 5 7 8 h 9 1 8 n j

9 2 8 4 7 5 0 3 1 9 6 0 3 0 6 1 7 4 8 5 3 9 2 6 8 2 4 0 1 8 8 7 4

k 5 h 6 g 0 f 8 d 4 s 1 a 2 q 5 w 0 r 3 t 5 y 7 u 5 p 7 a 3 z 8 p 0

16-Point Freeman Functional Near Field Chart

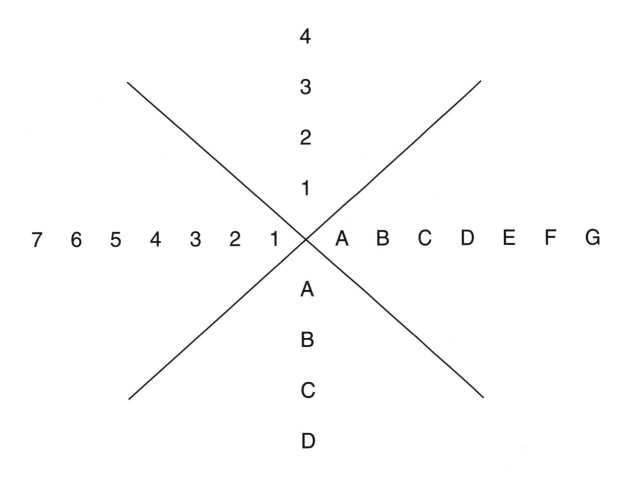

12-Point Freeman Functional Near Field Chart

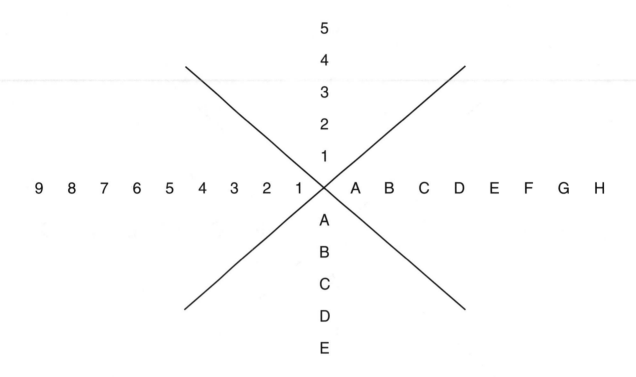

8-Point Freeman Functional Near Field Chart

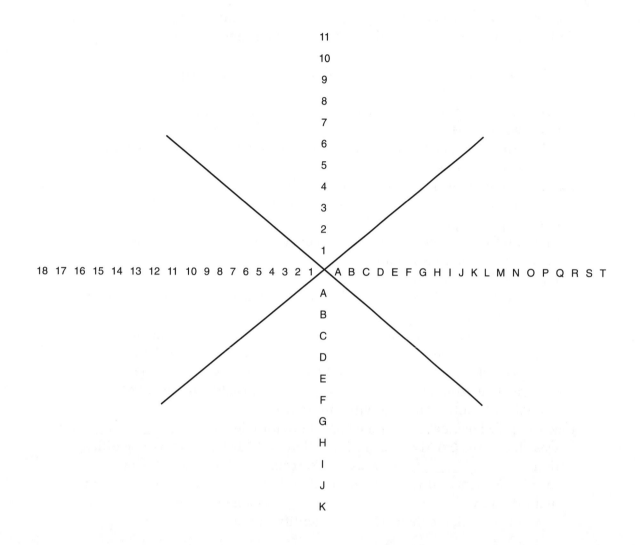

Form 2.4a (on letterhead)

Follow-Up Letter 1

Dear Dr. _____:

    I recently saw your patient, _____, on _____.
Following are test results obtained at that appointment:

    Snellen visual acuities at distance with present lens prescription:
      OD 20/200, OS 20/200, OU 20/200
    Metric visual acuities at 16 in. with present lens prescription: OD 4 M,
      OS 4 M, OU 4 M
    Amsler grid testing at 13 in.: OD metamorphopsic, OS metamorphopsic,
      OU metamorphopsic
    Confrontation fields at 1 M: OD full, OS full
    External evaluation: Eye movements full but hesitant in all quadrants of
      gaze. Pupils responsive to light.
    Standard refractive findings: Presently conventional lenses will not alter
      distance or near visual acuities.
    Tonometry: OD 18, OS 18
    Internal evaluation: Early nuclear changes, hazy media, 0.2 C/D, drusen in
      both eyes
    Low vision device evaluation: Distance—with a 4× galilean or keplerian
      focusable telescope, _____ was able to see 20/50 with a
      struggle with both the right eye and left eye; Near—with an 8× (16-in.
      standard) microscope, _____ was able to see 0.8 M print
      and 0.37 M continuous text with either eye.
    Electro-optical evaluation: With a closed-circuit television, _____
      was able to see 0.8 M text at 16 in. with a +2.50 D lens and 5× magnifica-
      tion. _____ was also screened with the Low Vision
      Imaging System and was able to see at both distance and near with mini-
      mal difficulty. _____ was able to appreciate a change
      in contrast, which enhanced his/her ability to see.

Impressions and Recommendations: Based on these findings, I am going to begin an
in-office and home rehabilitation program for _____ working with
his/her primary goals, specifically _____ and _____.
Each device is explored fully before its prescription is recommended. Should the
patient find a device inappropriate, we will test alternatives. Each system has some
advantages, but there are also some limitations that our patients must become familiar
with before the ultimate prescription.

    I hope this information is helpful to you. As we prescribe these systems, I will be
sending you updates. Thank you for allowing me to share in the care of your patient.
If I can answer any questions, please feel free to contact me at your convenience.

    Sincerely,

Follow-Up Letter 2

Date:
RE:
Dear Dr._____:

Per your referral, your patient, _____, was seen at the Low Vision Center for a consultation visit on _____. As you know, _____ is visually impaired due to _____ . Our intake indicates this impairment has created a handicap for _____ in the following areas:

1.

2.

3.

These were the issues addressed at this consultation visit. Today's examination indicated the distant acuities to be

OD: _____

OS: _____

Chart used: _____

At near, the best corrected acuity is _____ in the better right/left eye. Color vision is abnormal/within normal limits as tested by large-disc D-15. Contrast sensitivity screening indicates that contrast will/will not be a significant limitation to the successful use of low vision prescriptions. Binocular vision tests show this patient to be monocular/binocular/biocular at distance and monocular/binocular/biocular at near. The response to optical intervention was excellent/good/poor at distance/near/distance and near.

Based on today's evaluation, _____ has a poor/guarded/good/excellent prognosis for optical intervention and vision rehabilitation services. Appropriate appointments/follow-up contacts will be initiated by my office. I will keep you informed of all our interactions with your patient.

I appreciate your referral of _____ to the Low Vision Center and thank you for allowing me the opportunity to share in your patient's vision care. If I can answer any additional questions regarding _____, please feel free to call me at the office.

Sincerely,

Form 2.4b

Consultation Report

Date:
To:
From:
Patient:

Visual impairment/Dx:	Severe field constriction secondary to brain surgery.
Distant low vision acuity:	OD 10/10 (20/20)
	OS 10/10 (20/20)
Near low vision acuity:	0.8 M (magazine) at 35 cm OU; 0.5 M (newsprint) at 15 cm OU.
Binocularity:	Poor binocular function with present prescription.
Near device:	+2.00 D add with prism and cylinder—increases stereo or binocular function.
Glare/photophobia:	May need filters for outdoors, especially driving. Will evaluate with driving training sessions.
Visual fields:	Reduced to binocular fields of 85–105 degrees, right hemianopsia.
Prognosis:	[ ] excellent [ ] good [X] guarded [ ] poor

Recommendations/remarks: The recommended near prescription will alleviate much of her discomfort for long-term near tasks, such as reading and studying. The loss of peripheral fields has made it more difficult for her to maintain binocular vision at near. This prismatic correction does provide better alignment and stereopsis and will increase her periods of comfortable reading. Unfortunately, her major concern was obtaining a driver's license. She has a lot of emotional energy resting on the ability to drive. She was very upset when I told her she did not qualify for a routine licensing procedure with her field losses. There is, however, some chance we may be able to get a waiver if we follow some prescribed training and behind-the-wheel experience protocols. While the fields do not qualify her, they are modestly impaired, and we may be able to help her with prisms, special mirrors on the car, and behind-the-wheel training so she can safely operate a motor vehicle and pass a performance road test for the Department of Public Safety. I am requesting an extended revisit for her at the clinic to assess prisms for peripheral vision viewing. I am also requesting funding for her to be evaluated by a certified driving instructor who is a specialist in working with the visually and physically impaired in drivers' training programs. The instructor will need a 2-hour evaluation to determine this patient's potential for driving and provide an estimate of the amount of behind-the-wheel training she will need to become a safe, proficient driver. The instructor can provide a good estimate at that time of the cost of the complete driver's training program. Through this combined effort, we can help this patient realize her goal of being able to drive and live the independent and productive life she so strongly desires. If I can answer any additional questions regarding the proposed treatment and rehabilitation program, please feel free to call me.

Progress Report

Date:
To:
From:
Patient:

Comments:
I saw this patient at the clinic today for the evaluation of Fresnel prisms as a means of improving her awareness of objects in her right field of view. The prism field–awareness system can be of assistance to her in compensating for the field loss for both mobility and driving. She adapted quite well to the prism in the clinical setting and outdoors in a mobility assessment. I am recommending that this treatment option be pursued in conjunction with her driving instruction. The needed authorization request is attached. Her new lenses were dispensed today. As before, she is able to read newsprint comfortably. Her stereo acuity continues to improve.

Continuing our discussions about the driver training: I am having information about the behind-the-wheel training program forwarded to your office. The instructor works with the Rehabilitation Commission and was in charge of the drivers' training program for the Institute for Rehabilitation and Research. As you know, this is one of the most prestigious rehabilitation centers in the United States. As indicated in earlier letters, this patient does not have the visual fields to meet the criteria for driving set by the Department of Public Safety. Thus, I need this behind-the-wheel evaluation to ascertain her ability to compensate for the field loss with prisms and special car mirrors while operating a motor vehicle. This is the most professional and safest way to make a judgment on her ability to drive without endangering herself or others. This program is one of a handful in the United States, and we should take full advantage of its proximity. Driving is vital to those who are visually impaired and aspire to independence. In addition, it will enable the patient to be upwardly mobile when a job is obtained. The visually impaired are significantly handicapped in competing with their sighted peers in any job situation if they do not have access to private transportation. This patient has a great future and I want to do everything in our power to make sure she is able to reach her potential. If you need further information about my recommendations, please feel free to call me.
Authorization Request:

1. Fresnel prisms for field awareness system
2. Extended revisit for training with prisms (00505)
3. Authorization for 2-hour behind-the-wheel assessment of driving skills.
   Send authorization to Driver Rehabilitation Service.

The behind-the-wheel evaluation will provide the information as to whether she is a candidate for driving and, if so, how much additional training she will need and/or what kind of modifications will be needed for the car. The instructor will also be able to evaluate the spectacle prism system and its effectiveness in helping with her driving.

3 | After the Initial Examination

The following materials are given to a patient after the first consultation and examination. These materials reinforce what was covered in the office visit and provide activities for the patient to practice between visits. Although this information is given to the patient, the individual who brought the patient may have to read it. This includes family members in the rehabilitation process. Two sample letters that communicate the results of your examination and evaluation to referring physicians were noted in Chapter 2 (Form 2.4).

Many patients expect to receive a pair of glasses after the first visit and may be disappointed that glasses were not prescribed. In most instances it is in the patient's best interest to schedule another appointment for a confirmation of findings and training. Extending this initial, possibly emotional, visit can cause the patient to become fatigued, reducing performance and negatively influencing success. Scheduling a second visit will give the patient a break that includes training activities to do at home. This break with home training will not only make the patient a better candidate for optical intervention but will also show the patient how active his or her involvement in the rehabilitation process will be. These assigned at-home training activities will make most patients feel that something has been accomplished at the conclusion of the first visit, even if it is not obtaining the glasses they often anticipate.

CONTENTS

FORM DESCRIPTIONS

3.1 Available Community Services

Form 3.1 lists community resources that provide help to the visually impaired. Although not an exhaustive list, this information gives examples of the types of services you need to be aware of for the patient's benefit. You will have to seek out specific agencies and organizations that provide these services in your area and amend this list. The more active you are in the total rehabilitation process, the more the patient will benefit. You will be able to add to this list as you become more involved in low vision treatment. It is best to also include a paragraph about each organization and service. The information will also serve as a resource for your staff.

3.2 Materials to the Patient

Form 3.2 is a checklist of forms that should be given to the patient. You can add to this list as necessary. Note that you may need to contact some of these agencies to get the appropriate forms. This form is an important part of your patient record: It indicates the totality of care provided by your office.

3.3 Your Journey Begins

The proposed examination sequence consists of three or more visits. As described in Chapter 2, the first visit is a consultation and diagnostic visit to determine the extent of the patient's impairment. It is also the patient's first exposure to optical and nonoptical devices. After this visit and before you begin training with low vision systems, the patient may need a realistic pep talk. Form 3.3 reinforces the concepts discussed during the initial examination and should be given to the patient after the first visit. It may have to be read to the patient.

3.4 Helping You See Better

Some highly motivated individuals can manage, unwittingly, to train themselves to use their remaining vision. Even as their vision becomes increasingly impaired, they learn to make the best of their remaining capacity to observe critical details and shapes that help identify particular letters and numbers. They are able to pick up more information through their peripheral vision as their central vision fails. They learn to fill in letters, words, and even phrases they cannot actually see, like a detective using a few vital clues to reconstruct a crime. They also learn how to use the information they receive from their other senses to supplement the reduced amount of visual information. More important, they become confident in making judgments based on these minimal cues.

Not all patients succeed in learning these techniques on their own. The information in Form 3.4 focuses on encouraging patients to become aware of remaining vision and suggests techniques to optimize their vision. These activities should be completed at home before the second visit and are designed not only to help patients become more visually efficient but also to keep them actively involved in their own rehabilitation. *Note that these activities, as most of the others, are for patients with central sight loss.*

3.5   Additional Activities to Do Between Visits

Form 3.5 should also be given to the patient (with Forms 3.3 and 3.4) after the initial consultation and diagnostic visit. Form 3.5 contains a series of home exercises for patients to complete without optical devices and will introduce patients to motor tracking skills at close working distances (specific to head-borne devices) and techniques for using telescopes at a distance. The handout gives the patient continued contact with your office between the initial and second visits, when you will loan the patient optical prescriptions to begin active vision rehabilitation.

3.6   Certificate of Legal Blindness

Form 3.6 documents legal blindness. This is proof of entitlement to certain benefits. The form must be written on the doctor's letterhead. Each patient who qualifies typically needs a new form each year, especially for the Internal Revenue Service.

Available Community Services

Alcoholics Anonymous
Blindness and Visual Services (vocational rehabilitation)
Child Guidance Center
Community Health Nursing Services
Department of Health and Human Services
Departments of Social Services
Educational Services Centers
Family Outreach Centers
Family Service Center
Handicapped parking information
Head Injury Foundation
Health Department
Home Health Care, Inc.
Library of Congress (books on tape)
Meals on Wheels
National Association for Parents of the Visually Impaired
National Association for the Visually Handicapped
Psychiatric hospitals
Senior Citizens' Taxi Program
Senior Health Program
Sheltering Arms
Taping for the Blind
Transportation services
Veterans Administration
Visiting Nurses Association
Voting Assistance Hotline

Materials to the Patient

Information/Comments	Date Given to Patient
Certificate of Legal Blindness	
Amsler grid	
American Diabetes Association Membership	
Radio information services	
Large-print materials	
Telephone (free information)	
Outreach	
Macular Degeneration Association	
Retinitis Pigmentosa Association	
Transportation services	
Books on tape	
Catalogue for Nonoptical Aids	
National Organization for Persons with Albinism and Hypopigmentation	
Council for Citizens with Low Vision	
National Association for Parents of the Visually Impaired	
Other	

Your Journey Begins

The easiest segment of your journey to discover and optimize your remaining vision is complete. Through this initial comprehensive low vision evaluation, you and I were able to determine that you have useful sight that can be optically maximized. Now the hard part of the journey is about to begin.

Why will this part be difficult? You are going into unfamiliar territory, which can (and usually does) produce some anxiety. This anxiety can cause frustration. At times you may be angry or depressed. These feelings and thoughts are normal, because they are your way of coping with the work you are about to engage in. As you make this journey, you may decide to quit, but at least you now know you have options and alternatives for seeing. The phrase, *"nothing can be done to help you improve your sight,"* no longer applies. You can be helped with optical prescriptions. As you travel this new path, you will have to decide whether the energy and time you spend will be worthwhile. If you feel the time and energy will not be productive for you, you should stop.

Although you are unique, others have been in similar *visual* circumstances—each having made the decision whether to continue. Most, however, end up feeling better for having gone this far and develop personally satisfying "new ways of seeing."

You are the one who can make this choice. You are in charge.

GUARANTEES

What are your guarantees on this journey? There are no guarantees or promises except that it will take time to accomplish the things you want to do visually. To decide what you want, you will have to set goals. Take the time right now to list your goals. During the course of your training, however short or long, you will see the relevance of what you are doing. Although I cannot guarantee success, as a low vision specialist, I have worked with people like you and helped them achieve their goals through knowledge of the disease and functional implications of the eye condition that has created the vision problem. My staff and I will also help you set new goals as we work together.

STRUCTURING YOUR GOALS

Meeting your goals will require you to be flexible. The adjustments you make will be based on many factors, including your philosophy of life, values, and beliefs. Remember to keep your goals reasonable and recognize that small steps are going to be significant in achieving your ultimate goal. Also remember that if you do not see the relevance, it is time to stop and change direction or choose alternative methods of reaching your goals.

It is important that you feel in control of what you are doing—that you are the master of your visual destiny. You are the coordinator, and the outcome of the journey depends on your motivation, desires, and goals.

WHAT IS IN IT FOR ME?

Only you know how you feel. Your situation is unique not only because of your eyes but also because each of us is different. I have mentioned repeatedly that the work you will be doing is tough. When you accomplish tasks with your low vision device, feel proud. Realize that it is not necessary to like this new method of seeing, but to accomplish your goals you will have to be flexible and make changes in the way you see. Remember that you are still the person with all the traits you had before your visual difficulty, and you will be that person for the rest of your life.

SUPPORT FROM OTHERS

Coping with a visual difficulty can be easier with support from family, friends, doctors, and any other people important in your life. *Support does not mean "doing for you,"* but rather understanding your difficulties and being available when necessary. Remember, those who support you will be there when you need them. They, just like you, should maintain life as usual so that undue stress is not created for anyone. Try to remember that your life was balanced among different activities before your visual difficulty. Now you should try to achieve that balance again.

Even with support it is important to be an advocate for yourself. Do not be afraid to speak up—be assertive when it comes to letting people know what will make life easier for you. Doing so will make it easier for others to communicate with you. Your impaired vision does not make you any less intelligent, just more reliant on others for some activities.

A FINAL NOTE

The work we share in getting you back on the path to usable vision is a specialty. That is why you were referred here. Once we are done, you will still need routine and continued care for your eyes. If you have other medical problems, they should be monitored as well. It is important that you maintain a relationship with all your regular doctors—ophthalmologist, optometrist, internist, and others.

Finally, as far as your eyes are concerned, no one can be sure how long your vision will remain stable. Some people experience a vision loss and stabilize for the rest of their lives, whereas others experience a series of vision losses over time. Therefore, it is important to monitor your vision and consult your family eye doctor if you notice a change. When you have been told that those services have gone as far as possible, a phone call to us is appropriate. We will be here when you need us.

Helping You See Better

This information is designed to help you view around blind spots or areas of decreased vision. These suggestions should make things a little easier for you in your everyday experiences.

SCANNING

If you have ever seen a celebrity at a party or a powerful executive at a business meeting, you have seen the technique of scanning in action. A famous actress would never walk into a room and focus only on the person standing in front of her. Instead, she glances in all directions, checking to see who is there, who they are with, and whether they notice her entrance. Good drivers also use scanning. In addition to looking at the road directly ahead, they often look off to the sides, checking for a car that might emerge from a driveway, a person in a parked car who might suddenly open the door, and traffic flow at the next stoplight.

Scanning is a dynamic technique. People with vision loss can use it to pick up information they cannot obtain by looking directly at people or things. They see best by looking out of the corners of their eyes, and the continual eye movement of scanning helps them do so. This type of scanning can only be used if side vision is still available.

ECCENTRIC VIEWING

The static version of scanning is viewing an object by looking out of the corner of the eye. This is called *eccentric viewing*. A pitcher who appears to be looking directly at home plate but is really watching the runner at first base out of the corner of his eye is using eccentric viewing, as is the teacher who looks at the blackboard while checking on two students passing notes in the back of the classroom.

PRACTICE

Learning to view eccentrically is a little more difficult than learning to scan, so it is a good idea to practice while you are sitting in a familiar room. Try to look at an object right in front of you: a vase of flowers, a picture, or the face of a friend. It will probably appear blurry, or even invisible, erased by the blank spot in your central vision. Move your eyes to the left and right, up and down, until you find the angle that gives you the clearest picture. You might also try moving the object closer to your eyes, or farther away, to initially establish the best distance for viewing.

Once you have learned the best angle and distance, you can use them to locate other objects in the room. At first, eccentric viewing may seem strange, but with practice, using that angle will seem more natural. You will find that you are seeing much more than you thought possible.

After you know this angle, practice using it until you use it consistently. Now combine this with scanning. Here are two activities that may help:

1. Slowly roll a brightly colored tennis ball back and forth with someone. Use your eccentric vision to track it as it comes toward you and moves away from you. This also helps with eye-hand coordination.

2. Practice while sitting in a restaurant or shopping mall. Pick out a person walking by and use your eccentric viewing angle so that you see the person's head as clearly as possible and visually follow that person.

Practice will help you learn to do things more quickly and easily.

The next step is to practice eccentric viewing while you are moving around. It is best to begin in a familiar environment where the lighting is good. It may be very difficult at first because we typically walk in the direction our heads and eyes are pointing. Initially you will probably veer off to one side rather than walking in a straight line. Your old way of walking was learned over years of repetition, so it may take a while to learn this. But practice will pay off and you will soon be walking confidently at the same time you are using eccentric viewing to see all around you.

Using eccentric viewing also calls for relearning your old habits of eye-hand coordination. At first you may find it hard to reach for something when you are looking at it out of the corner of your eye. Practice with an unbreakable object on a nearby table. Sight the object with eccentric viewing and then reach for it. Noticeable improvement should come in only a few practice sessions.

These exercises are designed to foster a new relationship with your environment. Rather than confronting things directly, where your central vision can offer very little help, approach your environment from a different angle, using scanning and eccentric viewing. Your side vision will provide the visual information you need.

Eventually, you will learn the exact size and location of the blank spots in your vision. Then you can shift that blank spot away from the area you want to see. It is best if you can move the blank spot above or below the object you want to see.

OTHER SUGGESTIONS

- Learn to read body language rather than facial expressions. Perhaps you can no longer make out the minute changes in expression around another person's mouth or eyes, but you can still detect telltale body movements—for example, a tapping foot indicative of impatience, crossed arms that signal a lack of openness, or a posture that leans toward the speaker and indicates agreement.

- Try writing without looking at the paper. Your hands have learned the habit of writing and will probably continue to write legibly if you concentrate on remembering how to write rather than on trying to see what you are writing. Visualize the words in your mind. For guidance in keeping the lines straight, you can buy paper with raised lines that you can feel with your hand or paper with heavy black lines that you may be able to see.

Your doctor may provide some additional home training activities to do in conjunction with these exercises. Each activity will reinforce the others and help you make more efficient use of your remaining vision.

A final note on these activities—practice. You will have to unlearn habits of seeing that you have spent a lifetime forming: the way you look at the pavement when you walk, the way you hold the newspaper to read, the way you turn your head to look at something that catches your interest. You began learning these patterns as an infant and reinforced them with a lifetime of practice. Expect it to take *at least* a few months to teach yourself new habits.

Additional Activities to Do Between Visits

Because the lenses we usually use are unconventional, they will probably require the following:

1. Learning to readjust the distance between your eyes and the object of focus
2. Learning to view through a smaller field than you are accustomed to

Between now and your next visit, try a few activities at home that will acquaint you with some of the adaptations you will have to make with the lenses.

FOR NEAR

1. Every time you think of reading, writing, sewing, or any close activity, bring both hands approximately _____ inches from your face. Get your muscles accustomed to this distance rather than the 13–16 inches you have previously used for doing close work. The more you teach your muscles these memory skills, the easier it will be to use your lenses for close work.
2. With your hands at the approximate distance noted above, move your hands simultaneously from side to side. Imagine that you are reading or sewing. You will no longer move your head or eyes. Your eyes will remain stationary as your hands move the imaginary page.

Over time you will learn techniques suitable for you. These techniques will help you develop the ability to scan an object at close range.

FOR DISTANCE

1. Curl your fingers as if looking through a spyglass, put that hand up to your better eye, and look through it. Move your head around with this

simulated telescope and try to locate objects. This will acquaint you with the opening size and visual field you will be using.

2. Repeat the above procedure with the tube from a paper towel roll. Also try to follow moving objects with this simulated telescope.

Certificate of Legal Blindness

I hereby certify that I have examined _____ on _____ and know him/her to be blind within the meaning of the definition set forth below.

Definition of Blindness

The term *legally blind* describes an individual (1) whose central visual acuity does not exceed 20/200 in the better eye with correcting lenses, or (2) whose widest visual-field diameter subtends an angle no greater than 20 degrees.

(Code section 25 [b] [1] [c] of the Revenue Act of 1948)

Signature: _____ Date: _____

4 | **Treatment Options**

THE SECOND AND SUBSEQUENT VISITS

During the second visit, acuities can be re-evaluated and verified, and more in-depth visual field testing can be performed, including repeated Amsler grid testing. Refraction can also be repeated, especially when a patient has diabetes, is a child, or has multiple disabilities. Any test that yielded questionable results can be repeated.

Occasionally, tests need to be repeated to compare morning and afternoon visits (see Form 4.1), especially with reading lenses of +8.00 D powers and below. This almost natural range for near vision must be demonstrated again to reinforce the concept of a shorter-than-usual working distance. It will enable the patient to think about adapting to the shorter working distance. For most other patients, however, the majority of time at the second visit (see Form 4.2) will be spent selecting a tentative optical device to address the patient's needs and give him or her an opportunity to use the device in a number of practical applications (e.g., reading, writing, seeing bills, sewing, or viewing distant targets).

The devices described in this chapter are categorized into microscopes, magnifiers, telemicroscopes, telescopes, and electro-optical systems. This information is intended to help you understand the functional characteristics of these systems rather than prompt you to try to memorize the thousands of available devices. It will also help you decide which device to try after another has been rejected (make sure the reasons for the rejection are known).

In-office training with an optical system should begin at the second visit to ensure that the patient understands the use of the apparatus and can appreciate both the *real benefits* and the *limitations* of the device. The purpose of in-office training is to make sure the patient has developed enough proficiency using the system that it can be prescribed or, typically, be sent home as a loaner. The patient must demonstrate the ability to use the device for training activities in the office if success is to be achieved with the loaner system in a home training program.

When you are comfortable with the patient's ability, home training exercises can be given (see Chapter 5). You will need a device from your inventory to loan and training materials to give to the patient. Additional visits will be necessary until the patient demonstrates competence and comfort with the loaned device. A final prescription can then be discussed based on the success of the training and goals achieved. Remember, even if a patient has more than one goal, address only one goal at a time to avoid confusion.

PRESCRIBING RATIONALE

Now that the initial examination has been completed, you must be able to use the data to determine an appropriate low vision prescription. Typically, at the point of the second examination or visit, the following things have occurred:

- The case history has revealed those tasks most important to the patient (i.e., goals)
- The acuity has determined the level of magnification necessary to see the detail of those tasks the patient has indicated a desire to do
- Visual field testing has indicated the presence of any scotomas that make it difficult for the patient to perform those tasks
- Binocular testing has dictated the need for a monocular or binocular correction
- Contrast sensitivity testing has indicated the need for special high-contrast materials and even suggested the design of better light-collecting optical systems—for example, full-field microscopes instead of half-eyes

- Refraction has indicated the need for cylindrical correction to be incorporated with the prescriptive lens and dictated the type of device used

The factors below are the functional optical characteristics to consider at the second visit when deciding which one of the hundreds of devices available is most appropriate for the patient. These can be summarized as follows:

- Magnification: How much magnification does the patient need?
- Field of view: Can the patient tolerate a restricted field of view and by how much?
- Work distance: How much of a work distance does the task require?
- Mobility: Does the patient need to be mobile while using the prescription?

Every optical system has its own advantages and limitations. These must be appreciated relative to the functional considerations listed above. The available systems can be summarized according to these five categories:

1. Telescopes
2. Microscopes
3. Magnifiers
4. Telemicroscopes
5. Electro-optical systems

Table 4.1 outlines the functional optical properties of the five categories of prescriptive devices. Understanding this chart will be invaluable in determining the appropriate system to work with in the training sessions and as a final prescription for the patient. The requirements of the patient's desired task are compared to the functional optical properties of the devices in each of these category areas. This approach will make it easier for you to *prescribe* low vision devices, not just *dispense* them. In addition to this information on functional optics, you must also be familiar with the optical properties of all these devices, as reviewed in Appendices B and C.

In addition, a number of nonoptical devices complement the optical prescriptions in the following ways:

- Provide greater comfort (e.g., reading stands)
- Enhance contrast (e.g., filter paper, typoscope)
- Reduce glare (e.g., sun prescription, visors)

Table 4.1. Optical System Advantages and Limitations

Device	Magnification needed	Field of view needed	Work distance required	Mobility required
Microscope	Practical in +8.00–+48.00 D; special doublets preferred in +32.00–+80.00 D	The full-field microscope provides the largest field of view for comparable magnification; half-eye or bifocal design will result in some loss of field of view, but will allow for mobility	Has the shortest work distance of any system for comparable magnification	Full-field design precludes mobility; half-eyes or bifocals allow mobility but reduce field-of-view advantage
Magnifier	2.5× is practical as hand magnifier; >5× (+20.00 D), use stand magnifier or pocket magnifier	The magnifier is a compromise between the large field of the microscope and the small field of the telemicroscope; the patient can adjust the work distance and field of view to suit personal comfort	Magnifiers allow a more normalized work distance and acceptable field of view for comparable magnification; this advantage dissipates at 8× magnification and above	Magnifiers are portable and do not interfere with mobility; acceptable for use in public
Telemicroscope	Practical only to 8× magnification (+32.00 D); can design as a binocular with cap for greater power	Provides the smallest field of view of all devices for comparable magnification	Has the longest work distance for comparable magnification; usually not a practical field of view at ≥6× with surgicals and/or bioptic design	Full-field design precludes mobility; surgical design allows for travel and mobility but severely reduces field

Telescope	Hand-held systems practical to 10×; bioptic design practical to 6×; >10×, consider binoculars	Not applicable; all are used for distance; a focusable telescope suffers a loss of field of view over the use of caps when used as a near telescope	As a distance device, a telescope has a small field of view; a bioptic will have the smallest field of the types of telescopes typically prescribed; hand-held systems provide a larger field of view; consider binoculars; fields ≤6 degrees are typically not practical; keplerian telescopes have a larger field of view than galilean	Full-field design precludes mobility, especially >2×; bioptic design, while reducing field of view, allows for travel, mobility, and even driving (where legally allowed)
Electro-optical	System is practical from 8–60×	For higher magnification, it allows a more normalized work distance; may need reading correction with closed-circuit television	The words moving across the screen give the patient an apparent larger field of view, as it allows for faster information processing	The system precludes mobility; materials must be brought to the system for magnification; there are some portable systems, but to date, they have not been very successful

You should contact all the distributors listed in Appendix F and become familiar with as many of these types of devices as possible. Remember, a 100-W light bulb can be as instrumental to successful reading as a $3,000 electro-optical system.

Telescopes

Telescopes can be prescribed as one of the following options (Figure 4.1):

- Hand-held telescopes
- Clip-on telescopes
- Spectacle telescopes
    Bioptic
    Miniaturized
    Full diameter
- Binoculars
- Contact lens telescopes
- Intraocular lens (IOL) telescopes

Telescopes are prescribed for tasks with a work distance of 10 ft or more.

Of the optical devices available on the market, telescopes have the smallest field of view for comparable levels of magnification. As a starting point, you should assume the need for 20/40 distant vision. Magnification is determined by dividing the denominator of the distance acuity by the denominator of the target acuity. For example, if the best corrected acuity is 20/200, the telescopic magnification needed is 200/40 = 5×. Telescopes are typically available in magnifications of 4× or 6×. (You can, however, get a 5× magnification from Designs for Vision, Ronkonkoma, NY.) It is usually best to start with lower power (e.g., 4×), as it will be easier to use due to a larger field size and will allow initial success. With a 4× magnification telescope, the acuity will only improve from 20/200 to 20/50 (200/4 = 50). If 6× magnification is used next, you can expect an acuity of approximately 20/30 (200/6 = 33). To begin any training or take an acuity, it is best to initially prefocus the telescope on the chart or object.

Functionally, a hand-held telescope provides an adequate field of view up to 10× (10 × 30). Remember that the shorter the vertex distance (the closer the telescope is held to the eye), the greater the field of view. Typically, a field less than 6 degrees is not very practical for most patients. Also, the greater the power, the smaller the field of view. Manufacturers compensate for this law of optics by making the telescopes larger. Thus, you can expect an 8× hand-held scope to be substantially larger than a 4× hand-held system with the same field of view. Because it is hand-held, mobility is not impaired

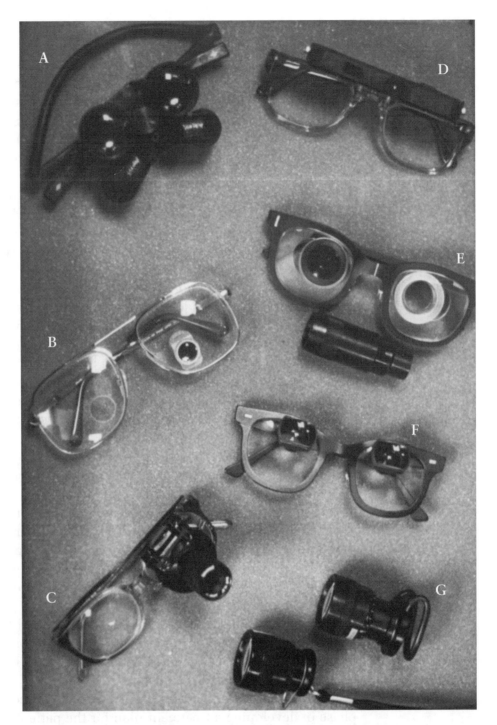

Figure 4.1. Telescopic prescriptions. A. The Beecher (Spalding Magnifiers, Houston, TX) is a head-mounted binocular system. B. The Behind-the-Lens (Optical Designs, Houston, TX) bioptic is a miniaturized telescope for better appearance. C. A hand-held telescope has a flip-up, clip-on attachment that can be used to attach it to the frame. D. The Ocutech bioptic telescope (Lighthouse, New York, NY) is a focusable bioptic system. E. The Designs for Vision (Ronkonkoma, NY) Expanded Field Telescope and Adjustable PD frame can be used for demonstrating the system to the patient. F. The galilean bioptic telescope is a fixed-focus bioptic system. G. A standard clip-on telescope and hand-held telescope.

with the telescope. Hanging the telescope around the neck can make it more convenient to use. The limitation of a hand-held system is that it requires one hand to be occupied during use. It is also inconvenient if it must be pulled out of a pocket or purse to be used. This inconvenience makes the device less likely to be used regularly. If a task requires two free hands, a bioptic telescope can be prescribed. This is a miniaturized telescope usually mounted in the upper portion of a spectacle carrier lens. While this type of mounting frees both hands, its miniaturized form noticeably reduces the field of view. It is sized for placement in the carrier lens of a regular frame. If a larger field is needed, however, this option can be made in a larger diameter telescope and mounted in the carrier lens as a full-field system. This allows the proper magnification, work distance, and field of view but now restricts the patient's mobility. The patient cannot look around the telescope for normal travel, and it is inefficient if the wearer's job requires mobility. To satisfy the demands for magnification, large field, and mobility, a clip can be placed on a hand-held telescope so it can be attached to a conventional prescription. All parameters can be met—correct magnification, work distance, and field of view. Mobility is facilitated by removing the clip or by flipping the telescope up and out of the way and using the regular lenses. Clipping the telescope to the glasses also frees both hands. The larger lenses also collect more light and are beneficial to patients with contrast sensitivity problems and eccentric fixation problems. Drawbacks of the system are a longer vertex distance, increased weight, and instability.

If, after all of these considerations, a still larger field of view is required, binoculars should be considered. These are physically bigger, so they have a larger field of view and better light-gathering capability. If both hands need to be free or the patient tires easily holding them, a tripod or lap pole can be used to hold the binoculars more comfortably for extended periods.

In summary, the rule of thumb is that hand-held telescopes are adequate to magnifications of approximately 10×, bioptics to approximately 6×, and binoculars to approximately 18×. This gives a wide range of magnification options for distant tasks.

The manipulation of the parameters of a telescope is the first phase of developing a treatment plan for the patient's distance needs. With a reasonable working knowledge of devices, you can effectively prescribe the appropriate system. Comparing these systems for similar tasks will also confer a better understanding of these functional optical parameters.

Two other types of telescopes are the contact lens telescope (high-minus contact lens with an aphakic spectacle prescription at approximately 20-mm vertex distance) and the IOL telescope. These systems allow limited magnification of 2× but enjoy a large field of view. The contact lens telescope requires the patient to move with constant 2× magnification (and spatial distortions). If developed, it is anticipated that the newer IOL systems will allow both telescopic viewing and pseudophakic viewing. The IOL system is still experimental and must be managed by the surgeon and low vision clinician.

Microscopes

Microscopes can be prescribed as one of the following options (Figure 4.2):

- Full-field microscope
- Executive/Ben Franklin bifocal
- Round segment bifocal
- Fresnel bifocal
- Half-eyes
- Uncorrected myopia
- Contact lenses
- Jeweler's loupe

Microscopes are appropriate for tasks that require work distances of 2–20 cm. They provide the largest field of view of all systems for comparable magnification, especially when prescribed as a single vision or doublet microscope. The field is reduced in the bifocal form of a microscopic correction but the design allows for some mobility. (One cannot walk around wearing a +20.00 D full-field microscope.) Obviously, the larger executive- or Ben Franklin–style bifocal provides a larger field of view but still makes mobility more difficult. A 22-mm round segment makes it easier to move about but somewhat difficult to localize through the microscope because of the small viewing area. If the patient has a desk job that requires little mobility, the Ben Franklin bifocal is probably the best choice. If the patient works in a stockroom and occasionally needs to see an invoice, the 22-mm round segment is the best choice. A compromise is the half-eye, which gives a larger field of view and, by sliding it down the nose, is easier to look over. As an added bonus, sliding the lenses down the nose also increases the magnification. An adjustable frame will allow a larger bifocal to be prescribed for people with mobility needs. The patient pushes the eyewear up to read and down to walk around, using a specially designed bridge.

There are other choices if the patient can tolerate a decrease in contrast. A Fresnel lens can be used and a large-field bifocal can be designed very inexpensively. A monocular contact lens providing +20.00 D of add is also possible. This gives a very large field of view and allows the patient to use eye movements (which are very limited behind a +20.00 D spectacle lens) to read. However, unless the

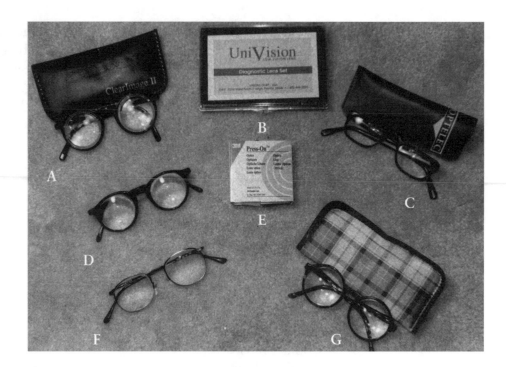

Figure 4.2. Microscopic corrections. A. Glass aspheric doublet microscopic ClearImage II lenses (Designs for Vision, Ronkonkoma, NY). B. Unilens Univision stick-on bifocal microscope (Unilens Corporation, Largo, FL). C. The Optelec (Westford, MA) prismatic half-eye system. D. Standard plastic molded microscopic hyperocular lenses. E. The Fresnel lens (Spalding Magnifiers, Houston, TX) can be used as a bifocal or full-field microscope. F. The Eschenbach full-field prismatic microscopes (Spalding Magnifiers). G. Volk microscopes (F/V microscopes).

patient is biocular and can use the other eye for distant and other tasks, this is not a practical application. Another interesting system is a reverse half-eye, used for highly myopic patients. It allows the patient to look under the myopic correction and enjoy a natural magnification (e.g., a −16.00 D myope enjoys 4× magnification at an approximate 6-cm work distance). Using the myope's own refractive error as a near prescription provides maximum contrast (no lenses to lose light). Another way to work with a myope is as follows. Correct a 20.00 D myope with a −12.00 D contact lens, leaving a +8.00 D add for reading. For distance, a −8.00 D spectacle prescription can be designed.

Remember, the decision of which microscopic magnification system to prescribe should be considered with regard for the magnification needs, field of view, and work distance requirements, as well as the importance of mobility to the task.

As a note, binocular corrections in microscopes are generally practical to a +12.00 D add. Prism is usually included (base in) with a standard half-eye to facilitate convergence. A full-diameter system also requires a prism and is very heavy unless a high-index material is used.

Finally, if a larger field of view than can be provided by a bifocal is needed and mobility is required, the full-field microscope is eliminated. If a significant distance refractive error exists, the half-eye microscope is eliminated. In this instance, a jeweler's loupe is the choice. A jeweler's loupe clips to the distance glasses and provides a full-field system. For mobility, the patient flips it up and walks with the distance correction. Sometimes the simpler the device, the better!

A brief review of magnification factors is in order. The power of microscopes is usually denoted in the D/4 system or using 25 cm as the relative standard distance. This means a +20.00 D lens provides magnification of 5× (20/4 = 5×). However, some of the new European devices use the formula D/4 + 1, which means a +20.00 D lens provides a magnification of 6× (20/4 = 5 + 1 = 6×). It is best if the clinician works with diopters or equivalent power to eliminate all confusion. If a patient sees 5 M at 40 cm, 1 M will theoretically be seen at one-fifth that distance, or 8 cm (40/5 = 8). At 8 cm, a +12.50 D add is needed for clear vision. (In this scenario, the +12.50 D lens is a 5× microscope.) If the patient sees 5 M at 25 cm with a conventional prescription, 1 M will be seen at 5 cm (25/5 = 5). This requires a +20.00 D add and 5× in this system is a +20.00 D lens. This exercise should make it clear why it is easier to work in diopters and centimeters.

Magnifiers

Magnifiers can be prescribed as one of the following options (Figure 4.3):

- Hand-held magnifier
- Stand magnifier
- Illuminated magnifier
- Fiberoptic magnifier
- Dome/bar magnifier

Magnifiers are a compromise between the longer working distance of a telemicroscope and the field of view of a microscope. Their disadvantage is that they do not allow hands-free use. Keep in mind that for any given magnifier the longer the working distance, the smaller the field of view. The patient will usually find a working distance that is comfortable and provides a reasonable field of view. Mobility is not a problem since magnifiers are not attached to spectacles. In addition, most of these magnifiers are portable.

Magnification is generally available in stand magnifiers and hand-held magnifiers to dioptric values or equivalent powers of approximately +32.00 D. Some of the stand systems are illuminated. If lighting or contrast problems exist, halogen or xenon lighting is

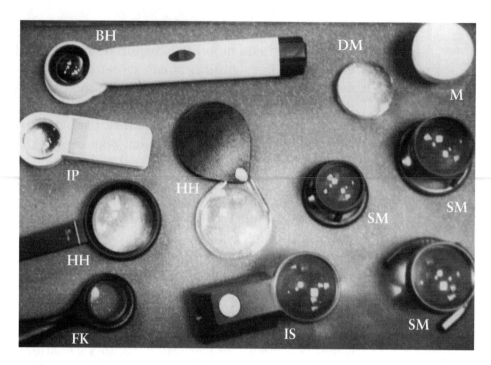

Figure 4.3. Magnifiers abound in the field and can be found as illuminated battery handle systems (BH), illuminated pocket magnifiers (IP), hand-held magnifiers (HH), dome magnifiers (DM), stand magnifiers (SM) (some requiring accommodation), and illuminated stand magnifiers (IS). The magnifier from the Freeman Kit (FK) using the Designs for Vision (Ronkonkoma, NY) doublet spectacle microscope is set in a handle to be used as a hand-held magnifier. This system provides high-quality imaging and usable field with higher levels of magnification.

extremely valuable. Above +32.00 D, the lens design is a pocket magnifier or a high-power stand magnifier. Both have a very small field of view and require the patient to hold the material very close to the eye. Remember when working with stand magnifiers that the power written on the box is usually greater than the effective power of the system when used by the patient. Also keep in mind that the aphakic or older patient must usually use a +3.00 or +4.00 D bifocal to obtain optimum magnification from many stand magnifiers. This is in contrast to a hand-held magnifier, which is held at the focal length of the system and should be viewed through the distance part of the patient's prescription. There are exceptions, and you must check with the manufacturer (or see Appendix C).

The equivalent viewing distance (EVD) classification system developed by Dr. Ian Bailey and his colleagues at the University of California, Berkeley, School of Optometry is the best reference system for the clinician to use when determining the true magnification of hand-held and stand magnifiers for the patient (Appendix C). The power of a magnifier is determined by the EVD. This is a practical and accurate way for the clinician to make sure the additional devices being evaluated will provide the same "magnification effect" for the patient as the initial treatment option.

Many patients will initially try to use the magnifier to obtain the largest work distance. However, with practice they usually find that as they bring it closer to the eye, the field gets larger and they can read faster. Eventually they use the magnifier at the spectacle plane. They often come back to your office wanting the power of the magnifier in a pair of glasses. You can now give them the microscope they initially turned down due to the short work distance. Magnifiers are often used as secondary prescriptions to complement microscopes. The microscopes are used for long-term tasks and the magnifier for more public, arm's length, short-term tasks.

Telemicroscopes

Telemicroscopes can be prescribed as one of the following options (Figure 4.4):

- Reading or surgical telescope
- Bioptic telemicroscope
- Clip-on telemicroscope
- Hand-held telemicroscope
- Binocular telemicroscope

Telemicroscopes are appropriate for tasks requiring intermediate work distances of 20–100 cm. The telemicroscopic design is essentially a distance telescope modified for near use by focusing for a near distance or adding of a plus cap to the objective lens. The focal distance of the plus cap dictates the work distance (+4.00 D cap = a work distance of 25 cm). The total power of the telemicroscopic system is the power of the telescope times the magnification power of the cap. In the 25-cm relative standard distance, a +8.00 D cap equals 2× magnification (D/4 = 8/4 = 2×). If we use a 4× telescope and add a +6.00 D cap (6/4 = 1.5×), the work distance is 16.6 cm and the total magnification is 6× (4 × 1.5× = 6×). A comparable microscope would be 24.00 D (4 × 6 = 24) as every 4.00 D equals 1× magnification in the D/4 or 25-cm relative standard distance system. A +24.00 D lens will have a work distance of 4 cm (100/24 = 4.16). This can also be determined by multiplying the power of the telescope by the diopter value of the cap to get the equivalent diopter value of a microscope. In our previous case, the 4× telescope with a +6.00 D cap will be equivalent to a +24.00 D microscope (4 × 6 = 24). Thus, the telemicroscope will increase the work distance from 4.0 to 16.5 cm and still maintain the 6× magnification required for the task. The disadvantage is the significant loss of field of view. The task and the patient's visual skills in compensating for the small field will determine its usefulness.

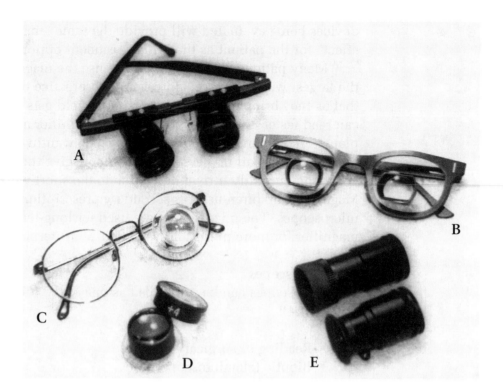

Figure 4.4. Telemicroscopic options. Most telescopes on the market are now focusable and will provide clear images as close as 8–12 in. (extending the tube focuses the system for near). A. Eschenbach Near Binocular telescopes (notice scopes converge) (Ridgefield, CT). B. Designs for Vision (Ronkonkoma, NY) surgical binoculars. C. New T-Specs or molded telescopic bifocals by Optical Designs (Houston, TX). D. Standard full-field Designs for Vision galilean telescope with a reading cap. E. A simple hand-held telescope can be focused for a near target by extending the housing.

The telemicroscope can be designed as a full-field spectacle or clip-on telemicroscope to try to improve the field of view. The larger the telescope, the larger the field of view. To this end, placing a cap on one side of a pair of binoculars and mounting it on a tripod for stability will provide a reasonable field of view and still maintain the needed magnification. For some tasks requiring a large field of view this is practical, for others it is not.

Surgical and reading telescopes have the telescope positioned in the lower or reading portion of the carrier lens. A surgical telescope has the cap built into the objective of the telescope; a reading telescope has a removable cap. Different work distances are created with different caps, which change the focus. A bioptic telemicroscope is a telescope mounted on the superior aspect of the spectacle lens to satisfy the patient's predominant need for distant viewing. However, the system can be focused for near, or a cap can be placed on the objective for a specified near working distance. This is a bioptic used as a telemicroscope and is prescribed when some intermediate viewing is required. The Ocutech Vision Enhancement

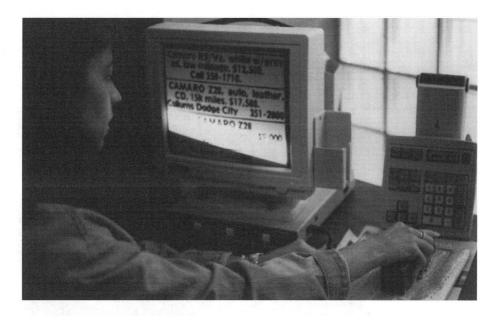

Figure 4.5. A large selection of closed-circuit television systems is now available. They provide high magnification with good contrast and comfortable work distances. They are available in several screen sizes, black and white or color, with hand-held cameras, built-in calculators, and connections for computers. See Appendix F for the various distributors.

System (Lighthouse, New York, NY) bioptic makes this process easier in the 3× and 4× powers with a self-focusing mechanism.

A clip-on telemicroscope is a hand-held telescope focused for intermediate distances. Its larger size provides a bigger field of view than does the bioptic. For very short-term tasks, the system can be hand held for convenience. A new type of telemicroscope, the T-Spec, that functions similarly to a bifocal with an extended work distance is available for low magnification needs through Optical Designs (Houston, TX). The telemicroscope offers good optics and an attractive cosmetic appearance.

Electro-Optical Systems
There are a few practical options in the electro-optical category:

- Closed-circuit television (CCTV) systems (Figure 4.5)
- Magni-Cam (Figure 4.6)
- Low Vision Imaging System (LVIS) (Figure 4.7) or V-max

A CCTV system is a unique device that requires some special attention as a prescription. It combines relative size and distance magnification features, requires either a reading lens or accommodation, and needs to be manipulated using an x-y table. A CCTV system offers an excellent field of view for close activities and maintains high contrast. Its disadvantage is that it is typically not

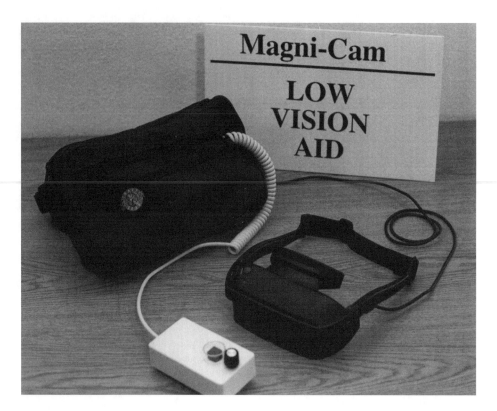

Figure 4.6. The Magni-Cam (Innoventions, Littleton, CO) consists of a hand-held camera that can be connected to a patient's television, a special high-contrast flat screen (as shown here), a heads-up display, or virtual reality glasses.

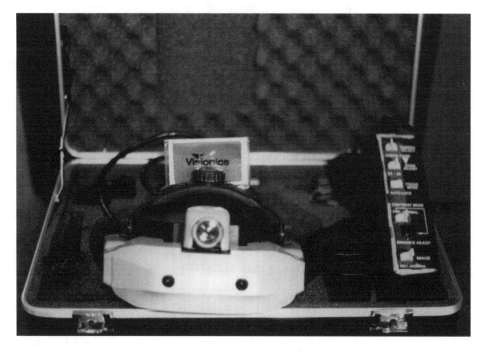

Figure 4.7. The Low Vision Imaging System (Visionics, Minneapolis, MN) is the epitome of high-tech low vision aides. It is a head-mounted display that uses on-board cameras for distant and near viewing. Its main feature is the ability to control contrast and optimize the image for each patient. It is focusable and allows limited mobility when being used.

portable, although some newer models make it easier to use one camera with several work stations. Newer models are also available that fit in a briefcase and project information on a 4 × 9 in. screen.

The CCTV system is a camera that focuses on reading material and transposes that material to an enlarged image on a television screen. The patient can easily get 20–40× magnification and still maintain a reasonable field of view and enjoy a comfortable work distance. This is an important option when older people with poor motor control or those with small fields are in need of high levels of magnification (8× or more). The reading material moves across the screen and the patient does not need to eccentrically view or track to process information. It is very effective, but be cautious when using it with younger children and students, as it does reduce learning some oculomotor and visual skills and makes it difficult for them to adapt to the more practical spectacle and hand-held systems they may need when they get older.

The Magni-Cam (Innoventions, Littleton, CO) is a unique electro-optical system that uses a hand-held camera that can transport the magnified image to the patient's television; a head-mounted display system (which looks similar to virtual reality glasses); or a small, flat, high-contrast, portable screen. It is easy to prescribe and demonstrate. Older patients frequently have some difficulty with the hand-held camera.

The LVIS (Visionics, Minneapolis, MN) (see Figure 4.7) and V-max (Enhanced Vision Systems, Costa Mesa, CA) are the most sophisticated electro-optical systems yet designed. They are heads-up display systems that consist of head-mounted cameras that project images onto the eye. Contrast and image enhancement controls allow each patient to adjust the systems for optimum viewing. They focus automatically and are currently the only electro-optical systems that can be used for distant and near tasks.

ADDITIONAL PRESCRIBING CONSIDERATIONS

In addition to the considerations just discussed, the clinician must give attention to the following secondary factors when prescribing:

1. Appearance of the system
2. Cost
3. Need for a refractive error correction
4. Availability
5. Stability of the disease

After all other factors have been addressed and you have found the perfect solution, any of the above factors can create havoc. Often the best optical prescription will be refused by the patient because of its appearance. This usually occurs with telescopes. Using more fashionable frames and tints will often help. The Behind-the-Lens telescope (Optical Designs, Houston, TX), the Designs for Vision Microspirals (Ronkonkoma, NY), or the Ocutech VES Mini (Lighthouse, New York, NY) are examples of smaller systems that are relatively hidden from view. Cosmesis is an important consideration for the clinician when determining an appropriate prescription. This factor is important for patients of all ages.

While costs are important, you should design the optimum system for the patient, demonstrate its benefits and limitations, and then discuss costs. Let the patients make the decision about how much they want to spend, not you: Do not look into your patients' pockets.

If a hyperopic or myopic astigmatic correction is needed, many stock devices will not be suitable. For example, if a high astigmatic error is present, this part of the prescription may need to be specially ordered. Also, if the patient is from another country and is leaving, waiting 4–6 weeks for a prescription is not an option. You may need to glue a cylindrical lens onto the optical system you want to prescribe to incorporate this cylinder. Availability is an important factor in your prescription or design consideration.

Finally, some vision conditions are of questionable stability. A diabetic, for example, may be considered fragile from a medical perspective. This should not interfere with prescribing a device, regardless of sophistication, if the device provides optimum visual function. If the eye has been relatively stable, a prescription for improved sight should be recommended. Discuss the prognosis with the patient. For some patients, good sight with an optical system for 2–3 weeks is worth the financial investment. Also, if a lower-powered system is introduced to the patient, it may be easier to adapt to a new, stronger device. It is important to prescribe a system that enables the patient to use his or her remaining vision, because the patient will be better able to use remembered skills should total blindness occur. The more visual memory a person has, the better concept development will be in a blindness rehabilitation program.

Field Expanders

The following are prescribing options for patients with severe field loss:

- Loose minus lenses (Figure 4.8)
- Reverse field telescopes
- Prisms (Fresnel or integral)
- Mirrors

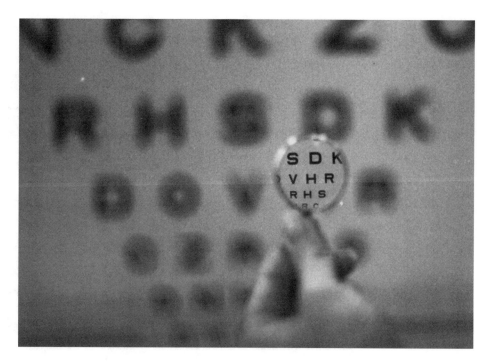

Figure 4.8. The simple concept of minification is shown by the use of a hand-held minus lens. The minification of the images provides the patient with reduced peripheral fields and more information about the area outside the restricted central field. Unlike the image in the figure, the image may be blurred for the patient.

These systems are designed to enhance field awareness, not to revitalize lost field. They are difficult to work with, as appropriate powers are usually found by trial and error and clinical judgment. These systems require extensive practice on the part of the patient, especially to establish environmental relationships.

A minus lens is typically used as a hand-held system positioned away from and in front of the user (see Figure 4.8). The minus lens minifies and compacts the environment so that more information is placed within the patient's constricted field. These systems should be placed out of the line of sight but such that they are accessible with minimal eye movement.

Reverse telescopes are similar to minus lenses and can be hand held or mounted in glasses. They are used by viewing through the wrong end (objective) of a low-power telescope. The telescope minifies the world, placing information within the patient's constricted field. These systems should be placed out of the line of sight but such that they are accessible with minimal eye movement. As an example, a 2.5× telescope creates a functional 2.5× minification. This means the patient can see 2.5 times more at one time but the detail is depressed 2.5 times. An acuity of 20/40 with spectacles is 20/100 through the minifier. It is used mainly as a spotting device.

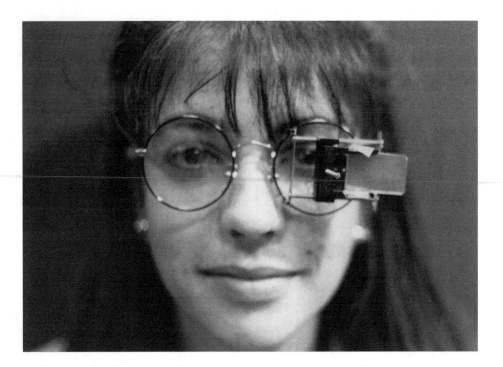

Figure 4.9. Field awareness systems using Fresnel or spectacle prisms are the most commonly used prescription for patients with peripheral field loss. The prisms are mounted laterally on the spectacle frame. With a small eye movement, the patient is able to see objects in the blind field. The Fresnel prisms provide more efficient access to the periphery because up to 30.00 D can be used. However, the image is usually very blurred. Ground-in or integral prisms provide good imagery but are only practical up to approximately 20.00 D. Shown in the figure is a research mirror prism (Optical Designs, Houston, TX) that provides the large displacement needed for efficiency and maintains a clear image for good acuity.

Prisms can be used with sector field losses or constricted fields of 10 degrees or less. They work by bending light, thus making information accessible to the usable portion of the retina. Typically, the prism is placed on the carrier lens over the field-loss side only, with the apex toward the center of the lens and positioned just out of the line of sight. This eliminates diplopia in primary gaze. For successful use, placement should be conducive to minimal eye movement. References related to proper placement of prism, as well as minifying lenses and reverse-field telescopes, are included in Appendix D.

Mirrors for field enhancement systems have not met with wide success because they obstruct vision and reverse the image (from left to right). However, some new mirror and prism systems from Optical Designs (Houston, TX) are showing promise (Figure 4.9).

Summary
The use of this prescribing rationale assists in the determination of an appropriate device for the patient and evaluation of that

device with respect to the requirements of the task and the functional properties of the optical system. As indicated earlier, the perfect prescription from an optical standpoint will not always be accepted by the patient, cosmetic appearance and cost being the most common reasons. In this case, evaluate other systems of equivalent power. Manufacturers' poor labeling systems make this a difficult task. The EVD classification system developed by Dr. Ian Bailey et al. can assist the clinician in determining the true magnification of magnifiers for the patient (see Appendix C). This type of work and scientific data allows clinicians a more "prescriptive" approach to low vision care rather than the "dispensing" approach found outside the clinical evaluation. Further experience in prescribing will come from working with additional patients, consulting with colleagues, and reading. Appendix D lists books and journals to help you stay current with developments in the field. The best advice is to have patience and be creative.

SUBSEQUENT VISITS

Once the patient has demonstrated reasonable competence with a device in the office, a loaned device and home activities (see Chapter 5) should be made available and the next office visit scheduled. Additional visits are necessary until the patient demonstrates confidence and comfort with the loaned device. The final prescription can then be discussed based on the success of the training and goals achieved. Even if a patient has more than one goal, address only one goal at a time to avoid confusion.

The length of time between visits can vary but 2–4 weeks is reasonable. Midway through that period, a staff member should call the patient to gauge the success of the home training. Form 4.3 will give the staff member guidance in questioning the patient and documenting compliance as well as progress in the home rehabilitation program. If at all possible, the person who works with the patient in the office should make the phone call because that staff member is familiar with the patient's personality. When the patient demonstrates competence on a subsequent visit, his or her own device should be designed and ordered.

Ordering and verifying low vision devices is no different than ordering and verifying any other optical or nonoptical system you dispense. The following checklist can serve as a guide in assuring that all the appropriate information has been gathered:

1. Verify all data before it is phoned in to lab.
   a. Power and type of system

b. Front vertex power of head-mounted microscopic systems when indicated

c. Frame

d. PD and bifocal height, when appropriate

2. The proper PD can be measured using any number of systems. For near systems, especially binocular systems, however, there is a calculation formula that can be used to adjust for the power of a microscopic system. Although many formulas exist, the authors have found the following by Dr. Ian Bailey to be the most easily used.

a. Obtain the distance PD in millimeters

b. Divide the distance PD in millimeters by the working distance in inches + 1

c. Subtract b from the distance PD. This will give you the calculated near PD

d. When ordering using this near PD, the lenses can be decentered appropriately, calculated with prisms by the laboratory, or both. For example, in a patient with a 60-mm PD and a +10.00 D microscope:

(1) working distance = 4 in.

(2) 4 + 1 = 5

(3) 60/5 = 12

(4) 60 − 12 = 48; near PD = 48 mm

3. The segment height should be determined based on the patient's preference and the power of the lens. Most often, the stronger the bifocal microscopic system, the higher the segment should be placed. That should make it less difficult for the patient to view through the optical center of the lens. However, this is only a guide, and the starting point should be individualized. Also be aware that the bifocal will create a blur scotoma inferiorly, possibly annoying the patient and making walking challenging. It sometimes makes sense for the patient to keep the original pair of glasses for general use, especially for near activities.

4. Proper power of the lens system, especially when using a head-mounted system, should always be determined in front vertex distance or calculated based on the actual lenses in the trial frame being used at that time.

5. All of this information should be verified before dispensing.

There is truly an art to dispensing a low vision device (see Form 4.4). After the device has been adjusted, the use of the device should once more be reviewed and the ergonomics of the system emphasized. Dispensing should be performed by a staff member first and then signed off on by you. Why? If, for some reason, there is a problem at the time of dispensing, the staff member has someone to turn to. You will then have ample time to think about your management options before meeting with the patient. If you were the entry-level dispenser and ran into problems, you would have no one to turn to and would have been caught off guard. This is simply good defensive practice management.

Your work is not done after the final dispensing. It is important to ascertain whether your services have helped the patient and if the devices dispensed are being used. A phone call or follow-up visit 1 month after dispensing is valuable. (Obviously, the patient should know that you are available before then, but you give the patient additional confidence in your work by indicating that you will follow up.)

Remember, the patient is also the referring doctor's patient, and your services should be consistent with a team approach, with the referring doctor as an integral part of general and routine eye care. Reports should be sent out after most visits.

When an optical system is dispensed, it may also be helpful to provide the patient with an information sheet on microscopes, for example, Form 4.5. You may also give the patient a form that provides refresher information on how to use the system at home (see Form 4.6).

FORM DESCRIPTIONS

4.1   AM/PM Refractive Error Check Form

The refractive error correction is often variable, especially for patients with diabetic retinopathy or central serous maculopathy. You may find a significant refractive error with improvement in acuity at the first visit. This may not be stable, however, especially when the patient reports fluctuation in vision. In these cases, it is best to recheck the refractive error correction at a subsequent visit before prescribing. If the first visit was in the morning, schedule the second visit in the afternoon and visa-versa.

4.2   Follow-Up Form

Two formats for record-keeping for the second and subsequent visits are provided. Using a standard form for all your subsequent visits leads to more consistent data collection and better patient evaluations. It also helps to ensure that all patients' optical and nonoptical goals are addressed.

4.3   Telephone Call Form

Patients can become easily frustrated with the home training exercises and activities. Having a staff member contact your patients by phone and inquire about their progress significantly increases patient compliance with the training program. In most cases, problems with the training can be resolved over the phone, without wasting further clinical time. Most important, it assures your patients that you and your staff are interested in them as individuals.

4.4   Dispensing Visit

The dispensing visit is a very important clinical interaction. Patient expectations are often very high and sometimes unrealistic. Not only must the prescription be fit properly at this visit but your patients must be reinstructed in the proper use of the devices. This includes reminders about proper lighting and good, comfortable posture. Taking this time during dispensing visits to provide additional instruction is time well spent.

4.5   Frequently Asked Questions about Microscopes

You cannot possibly anticipate all questions. Often what you believe patients know is unfounded. Providing an information sheet at the time of dispensing is valuable to your patients and is an excellent practice builder. You can make up such question-and-answer sheets for all of your commonly prescribed devices. These will reinforce your verbal instructions. Use this form as a guide.

4.6   Device Reading Hints

No matter how much you have discussed and demonstrated the close work distance, patients can forget what they have been told as soon as they walk out of your office. Providing this reminder sheet will reinforce your in-office instructions and make patients feel more comfortable calling you with problems. This can save you and your staff from the aggravation that arises when patients become frustrated because they are using systems incorrectly.

Form 4.1

AM/PM Refractive Error Check Form

Name: _____   Date: _____

Charges: Covered: _____

                 Noncovered: _____

Previous visit: AM/PM   Today's visit: AM/PM

Rx: OD _____ /VA _____   OD _____ /VA _____

     OS _____ /VA _____   OS _____ /VA _____

     Add _____   Add _____

Near only

     OD _____ /VA _____   OD _____ /VA _____

     OS _____ /VA _____   OS _____ /VA _____

Comments and additional tests:

Final Rx: OD _____   VA _____

                OS _____   VA _____

                Add _____   PD _____   Seg. ht.

Fee: Frame _____ Lenses _____ Additional _____ Total _____

        Name _____

Sun filters:

Recommendations:

Dispensing Instructions

Mail:

Called for dispensing:

Follow-Up Form

Name: _____   Date: _____

Subjective: How patient feels before treatment

Objective: Measurements, test results, examination observations

Assessment: Status of problem, progress of care, new problems

Plan: Prescription

Subjective: How patient feels after treatment

Subjective (before): _____

_____

Objective: _____

_____

Assessment: _____

_____

Plan: _____

_____

Subjective (after): _____

_____

Additional information: _____

_____

Subsequent Examination Visits

History

(Any Changes in Vision?   /   Training Progress   /   Today's Goals)

Acuity:

Assessment:

Visit summary:

Date: _____   Patient: _____

Clinician: _____   Accompanied by: _____

Telephone Call Form

Patient's name: _____   Telephone: _____

Information to be discussed:

1. Lighting   4. Reading materials

2. Work distance   5. Attitude of patient

3. Length of time (15 minutes) 6. Problems

Date: _____   Device: _____

                           Print: _____

Comments: _____

_____

Tone: _____

Date: _____   Device: _____

                           Print: _____

Comments: _____

_____

Tone: _____

Date: _____   Device: _____

                           Print: _____

Comments: _____

_____

Tone: _____

If the patient is unsure of the usefulness of the device after 4 months, the choice of device should be re-evaluated.

Form 4.4

Dispensing Visit

Patient's name: _____   Date: _____

Charges: _____   Deposit: _____   Balance: _____

Rx: OD _____ VA _____ Add _____ VA _____

OS _____ VA _____ Add _____ VA _____

Working distance: _____

Instructions:

Follow-up:

Signature of dispenser: _____

Frequently Asked Questions About Microscopes

Q.   Why can't I be prescribed a conventional pair of glasses?

A.   Because of your eye condition (e.g., macular degeneration, diabetic retinopathy, glaucoma), a conventional pair of glasses cannot be made strong enough for you to see small objects. For you to read, sew, write, and do other activities, it is necessary to use a microscopic lens that can be made strong enough to meet your visual needs.

Q.   Why do I have to hold the material so close to my face?

A.   You need to hold the material close to your face because of the optics of the microscopic system. The stronger the system, the closer the material must be to be clear. This is the only way your material will be clear.

Q.   Can I hurt or lose the only vision I have by using low vision devices?

A.   You cannot hurt your vision by using any type of low vision device. In fact, the more you use your vision, the more you stimulate the remaining vision.

Q.   Why is one lens frosted?

A.   Because of the nature of the microscopic lens you are working with, it will be virtually impossible to use both eyes together. As a result, one lens has been frosted (or taped). This frosting is designed to minimize visual distraction. This will eliminate confusion between clear images in the good eye using the microscope and the other eye behind the frosted lens. As you progress with the use of your lens, you may find that the frosted lens is not as beneficial as when we started. The frosted lens can be removed at any time and replaced with a clear or prescription lens. The frosted lens does nothing to impair or damage the eye that is not being used.

Q.   Will I ever be able to read as fast as I used to?

A.   All patients perform differently. Success in accomplishing goals depends on the level of motivation and desire to succeed.

Device Reading Hints

At today's visit you were given a prescription or training material. Below are some hints to help you.

From this point on, we are all in this together—partners in meeting your goals.

Do not try to overdo in the beginning. This can become tiresome and frustrating.

Remember, when you are using this device, start with your material close to your nose and then pull away until you can focus clearly on the material to get the best reading or working distance. *Good lighting is very important!*

Call if you are having problems. We are here to help you make the adjustment to using your device(s). If we cannot solve your problem over the phone, we will make an appointment for training.

Our number is _____. Ask for _____. If we are not in, please leave a message on the answering machine with your phone number. We will call you as soon as we are back in the office.

Thank you for being our patient and allowing us to help you meet your goals. We will do our best, along with your help.

5 | Low Vision Training

INTRODUCTION

Gregory L. Goodrich

The use of low vision devices goes far beyond the principles of optics. It is a challenge to encourage the use of low vision devices for several reasons, including the patient's level of motivation, frustration, confusion, and so forth.

Low vision training combines systems optics with functional activities; it allows the patient to systematically learn to perform with or without a device to enhance the use of remaining sight skills. Activities are typically designed to teach the use of a low vision device so that it becomes part of the patient's everyday visual processing. Activities designed to stimulate the use of remaining sight are similar to those designed for amblyopia therapy. Ultimately, the activities help an individual learn how to use remaining and enhanced sight so that it may be appropriately integrated into the sensory-motor system that remains intact.

Seeing the world around us is a learned behavior. From the time we are born, we learn to recognize and interact with the visual world. Each new situation requires new learning. In practice, however, this is manifested as applying prior learning to the new situation. In some cases in which the new situation is similar but subtly different from a prior learning experience, we find ourselves making predictable mistakes. For example, when people buy a new car they often find themselves reaching to the wrong place to turn on the headlights or windshield wipers. In the old car, the windshield wiper control may have been to the left of the steering wheel, while in the new car it is on the right. For a while they will reach to the left instead of the right when trying to turn on the windshield wipers. Gradually, they will make this mistake less often until they have learned the new position. Low vision devices make print look different: larger, closer, and sometimes higher or lower in the visual field. It will take time to learn to work with this "new" print, just as it takes time to learn where the windshield wiper control is in a new car. Practice and training help when learning to see the visual world with low vision devices.

Learning takes time. In general, the worse the patient's vision (measured as visual acuity, visual field, contrast sensitivity, binocularity, color vision, etc.), the more that patient will find training beneficial. With regard to optical devices, the stronger the system, the more training is appropriate. One caveat, however, is that for a given level of vision loss, **the patient who has had prior vision rehabilitation may need less training**.

Patients vary greatly in their abilities to adapt to vision loss. Motivation, cognitive plasticity, depression, family and social support, and many other factors (singly or in combination) play an important role. Still, it is important to give the patient an idea of what to expect during the course of training. The following thoughts should be helpful in this respect.

First, as you work with the patient during the examination and prescription process it will become evident how easily the patient adapts to new situations and how well the patient follows directions. Was there a struggle with even simple visual tasks or was there easy adaptation? Did the patient orient well to the examination room? Was walking in and out easy? Such observations help you form an expectation of how well the patient will adapt to training. As you become more skilled in low vision work, you, too, will learn, and your estimates will become more accurate. Do not, however, give the patient rigid estimates. Instead, use a range of training sessions or days with the low end of the range being what you think the patient will need and the high end being a very generous estimate. The rationale is quite simple; if the patient responds well to the low vision device and training, congratulating this remarkable progress is appropriate and builds confidence. If the patient responds slowly, you can tell the patient that good progress is being made as you expected and that continued effort is likely to produce additional gains. Do not forget to take into account factors such as poor motivation, lack of plasticity, depression, and so forth. If any of these seems to be present, add an additional week to your estimate and ensure that the patient has external support. This support can come from friends or family. It may also be helpful to have someone from your staff call the patient once or twice each week during the first few weeks. These phone calls are especially beneficial if the patient lacks outside support. Think of this as "just checking in," to remind the patient to use good lighting, good posture, proper working distance, and so forth. Obviously, the caller must be familiar with the patient and the device(s) being used.

When working with telescopic devices, the patient may require up to several weeks to become comfortable and competent. The time required ranges from a few days to 3–4 weeks of daily practice. For reading tasks, the patient can expect to see improvements (faster reading speeds) within a few days; however, this may be in the range of 10–15%. If the patient's initial reading speed is 30 words per minute, this is a gain of only 3 or 4 words per minute, and the patient may not have a sense of improvement. Only during accurate timing of a patient's reading will improvement be noted. Thus, you may caution the patient that initial improvements are likely to be modest and that it may take 2–5 weeks of daily practice before the best reading speed is achieved. Interestingly, reading duration improves at a much faster rate than reading speed. It is not uncommon for visually impaired patients to be able to read for at least 50 minutes with a closed-circuit television within the first week and for at least 20–30 minutes with optical devices after as few as 7 training days.

Patients with central field losses will, in general, have a slow but steady rise in reading speeds. If you plot reading speed on a daily basis, you are likely to see a line that rises slowly from left to right. Maximum reading rates may not occur until as many as 3–5 weeks of training have been completed. Patients with peripheral field losses will usually show a much steeper learning curve and may be expected to reach a maximum rate within 2–4 weeks. The patient may not show much improvement in reading speed the first 2–3 days of training and it is very important to ensure that the patient is not discouraged. If the patient realizes that training and practice can take several weeks, it will be easier for him or her to continue putting in the required effort. Patients who get the best low vision examination and device will still fail if they get frustrated too easily and give up. It is up to you to manage the training process to promote success.

There are other strategies that you should follow. A very important clinical philosophy is to use success-oriented strategies. Using these strategies you select training tasks that your patient is certain to perform, even though these may not match the patient's ultimate goals. For example, rather than starting distance training with the recommended 8× telescope, start the patient with a 4× or 6× using closer or larger targets. This allows the patient to take advantage of the greater field of view and slower apparent motion with the device while becoming familiar with using telescopes. Once proficient with the lower power telescope it will be easier for the patient to graduate to a higher power and success is more likely.

For reading tasks in which the patient's ultimate goal is to read smaller print—smaller than 1 M, for example—it may be better to start the patient with larger print and a low-power magnifier for the first few days or week of training. Once the patient has gained some degree of reading fluency, the power of the magnifier can be increased and the print size decreased. If the patient starts with large print (i.e., 1.6–2.0 M), it may be better to use an intermediate size for several lessons before dropping down to the final print size specified in the patient's goals.

You and your patients should recognize that visual tasks are complex. Reading, even for a normally sighted person, is more than simply "reading." It also involves identifying the material to be read. For example, when reading a newspaper, the reader must visually identify the material to be read and distinguish one article from the remaining print, pictures, and lines. In short, the reader must distinguish the "figure" from the "ground." Psychologically speaking, figure-ground recognition is one of the basic building blocks of reading (and many other visual tasks). Reading also involves identifying what is a "word." Usually, a word is defined by the space before and after it. Ifthespacesarenotpresentornotseenitisdifficulttoread (If the spaces are not present or not seen it is difficult to read). For many partially sighted individuals, particularly those with central field losses, the ability to visually define a word is difficult because the resolution of the peripheral retina is not sufficient for normal-size print, and even with eccentric viewing, the detection of the space between words is difficult. Increased magnification may be of little benefit, and the time required to relearn reading skills is usually considerable. The more patients understand why reading is difficult and how they can largely overcome the difficulty with patience, practice, and appropriate prescriptions, the more likely they are to succeed.

The training aspect of low vision care is often responsible for separating success from failure. The patient must become involved in specified tasks with the new prescription that will enable success. Like any other training program, the tasks must begin with the simple and build to the more complex. The following activities can be used for this purpose, in any order and sequence. Just as each patient is an individual, each sequence of activities for a patient should be individualized. It would be great if there were a cookbook approach to training a low vision patient but, in fact, each activity a patient wishes to accomplish has component parts, some of which the patient can perform and some of which the patient cannot.

Another aspect of separating success from failure is comanaging the patient, a critical concept in any intensive interactive program. Following are five thoughts to keep in mind as you proceed through each patient's low vision program.

Comanagement

1. Ability to give instruction
2. Ability to understand instruction
3. Attitude toward treatment
4. Opportunity to perform task
5. Perseverance to complete task

Note that the areas of responsibility are evenly divided: The ability to give instruction and the opportunity to perform the task are the responsibility of the doctor, whereas the ability to understand the instructions and the perseverance needed to complete the task are the responsibility of the patient and those who work with the patient. The area that is shared by you and the patient is the attitude necessary to be successful. Without a positive outlook, any program you put together will be fraught with difficulty. Review these concepts with your staff; they are important to a successful low vision practice.

Here are some general guidelines to follow when you interact with a patient using any optical system.

1. Establish the focal length of any system. This is critical because a slight deviation from the range of focus will cause the object being viewed to become blurry. For focusable systems, learning how to focus automatically is important for ease of use. The work distance will also affect the patient's posture.

2. Establish the usable field of view of the system. The lens diameter and the distance from the patient's eye will determine how many objects can be seen at one time. Unlike conventional eyeglasses, in which a whole scene or page might be viewed, the powerful low vision device may only be useful for picking up part of a scene or page. For example, if a microscope is to be used for reading, the amount the patient is able to see at one time determines the ease and speed with which he or she will be able to read. It may also determine the length of time the device can be used before the patient becomes fatigued (see Figure 2.3).

3. Establish environmental criteria, specifically for lighting. Regardless of the type of low vision device being used, correct lighting arrangement is essential. Too much light is just as bad as too little light. Improper placement of light can cause glare, shadows, and reflections that will decrease the effectiveness of a low vision device. The type of light used should also be considered (e.g., incandescent, fluorescent, halogen, or combination).

4. Each visit should begin with a review of the optical or nonoptical system being used and its advantages and limitations. Instruction for home training should take place in the office. Explain that these are training materials, vehicles to more functional activities such as reading and writing. Encourage family members or friends to listen carefully to the explanation, because they spend considerably more time with the patient and may be able to give valuable input at home.

5. At each visit, the goals of the patient should be reviewed. At times, these goals will need to be modified or the types of devices recommended will need to be changed.

6. To avoid confusing the patient, one device should be worked with at a time. This is not done because of the patient's age or intel-

ligence but rather to avoid overwhelming the patient with instructions and activities. By working initially with one device, one can ultimately establish a successful point of reference from which other options can be evaluated. Even if the initial device is ultimately not the device of choice, it will give the patient knowledge of what can be achieved.

7. A follow-up schedule should be instituted at the conclusion of your active involvement. The one that the author has found beneficial is a 1-3-6 month cycle. After 1 month, the patient is called and asked about any changes in vision. The questioning occurs again 3 months later. Finally, a 6-month follow-up visit is scheduled, approximately 11 months after the last face-to-face office interaction. This enables you to continually update information on the patient and communicate any changes in your findings with the primary eye care practitioner as needed. Additionally, patients are always told that, should they notice a problem, the low vision facility is the second call after their primary eye care practitioner has been alerted and has intervened. When the primary eye care practitioner decides that nothing needs to be done medically, the patient can return for an update or a modification of the low vision device.

The remainder of this chapter consists of instructions and homework handouts to give to the low vision patient. They should be assigned according to the patient's primary goal. Do not burden patients capable of reading or doing other near activities easily with these training materials.

CONTENTS

FORM DESCRIPTIONS

Directions to be given to the low vision patient are supplied in easy-to-read, 12-point, bold print.

5.1 Calendar

The calendar is a simple way for the patient to monitor individual feelings of success. This is helpful when the patient returns for follow-up care.

5.2 Low Vision Homework Instructional Materials—Near

The exercises in Form 5.2 are designed to be used specifically with loaned optical devices in a home training program and should be used in conjunction with the exercises in Forms 5.5 and 5.6. The instructions may have to be read to the patient. The materials are presented in 12-point type but you can enlarge or decrease the size of the materials to meet the individual needs of each patient. These activities can be used with any near system. They can also be used in the office for preliminary training and education in the use of low vision devices.

If steady fixation is a problem or poor eccentric viewing is noted (e.g., the patient skips lines and has poor sentence acuity versus single optotype acuity), the patient should be considered for eccentric viewing training tasks (Forms 5.3 and 5.4). Once the patient has mastered eccentric viewing, proceed to these home training instructional materials.

5.3 Eccentric Viewing I

The exercises in Form 5.3 are designed to make the patient conscious of eccentric viewing and proficient at maintaining off-foveal fixation. The specific material in these exercises must be understood thoroughly by the patient in the office. Therefore, you should demonstrate the activities in the office before assigning them for home training. The instructions on these pages may have to be read by someone other than the patient. Use patient feedback to help guide these activities. Be available by telephone to answer questions; this training is difficult. The exercises are offered in three type sizes:

16 point (Form 5.3a), 12 point (Form 5.3b), and 8 point (Form 5.3c). A printer will understand the point notation for type size should you want to vary the size of the print. To convert to M notation for consistency with your low vision evaluation, use the following approximate conversion formula: point size/8 = M.

Form 5.3d, Eccentric Viewing for Social Situations, is included here to emphasize the need for patients to use this technique while interacting in the community. These activities are designed to decrease the patient's uneasiness in social situations; they should be practiced until proficiency is achieved.

5.4 Eccentric Viewing II

Form 5.4 is another variation of eccentric viewing training that will help the patient apply the new eccentric viewing skills to different tasks and activities. Varying the exercises will also help prevent the patient from getting bored.

5.5 Low Vision Tracking Exercises

The low vision tracking exercises can be used to help the patient develop proficiency with a near-point device. The exercises can be read, used as a game to find certain letters or words, or used to improve saccadic eye movements and localization skills by jumping from one column to the next. The materials are not a magic solution for patients with an optical device. You must decide what oculomotor skill needs to be developed and use these materials to design a training program that will help the patient achieve this skill. This is truly the art (clinician) and practice (patient) of low vision. Be creative and have fun.

5.6 Proficiency Activities—Near

The activities in Form 5.6 encourage automaticity in the use of near devices. Each activity stresses application of the use of the device to a "real" situation. There is no specific sequence, as each activity trains the patient in a skill directly related to the use of the device. These activities are written for user-friendly home training application. In most cases you will need to provide the listed materials for the activity. Some must be performed in the clinic or office under doctor/instructor supervision.

5.7 Low Vision Homework Instructional Materials—Distance

The exercise instructions in Form 5.7 are the same as those in Form 5.2 except they are designed and modified for use with telescopes and electro-optical systems. The distance training materials concentrate on localization through a telescope; the patient must learn to find things through a small aperture. As with the other section, you may need to provide some of the materials for the activity. The instruction sheets are to be given to the patient.

It is usually easier for most patients to concentrate on one type of device at a time—distant or near. Make sure the patient has achieved optimum performance in the office before sending materials home.

5.8 Proficiency Activities—Distance

The activities in Form 5.8 encourage patient awareness of the limitations and uses of a telescope by encouraging automaticity much the same way as the near proficiency activities allow for practical use of those devices. These handouts are designed to be taken home with the patient but should be reviewed in your office before initiating a home training program. Some activities are better managed in the clinic or office.

5.9 Low Vision Homework Instructional Materials—Peripheral

The activities in Form 5.9 encourage the patient's awareness of the peripheral visual information that has been lost to disease or injury. The use of mirrors, prisms, minus lenses, and general viewing are covered. Whether a device is used before teaching scanning depends on your philosophy.

5.10 Proficiency Activities—Peripheral

The peripheral proficiency activities enable the patient to become efficient in using devices that take a passive system (peripheral) and make it active (central) for a moment. Most of these exercises should be performed in your office, at least initially. Provide the proper prescription and materials for these activities and ensure that the patient can perform them in the clinic before attempting them at home.

Calendar

Sunday	Monday	Tuesday	Wednesday	Thursday	Friday	Saturday

Low Vision Homework
Instructional Materials—Near

You have demonstrated readiness to work with home training activities. These activities are designed to help you relearn some reading skills. Reading is a complex perceptual and visual physiologic activity. It involves not only being able to see individual letters and words and track along a line, but also being able to use cognitive and perceptual skills.

These activities will start you on the road to visual tracking skills and letter, word, and number discrimination. Here are some hints to help you with these activities.

1. You should work on these home activities for no longer than 15 minutes at a time. This seems to be the appropriate amount of time one can initially work without becoming frustrated or uncomfortable. These 15-minute work segments should be done three times a day, 5 days a week. As you work, if you find that 15 minutes go by quickly and you are not having problems, increase your work time by 5-minute intervals.

2. During the 15-minute segment, ensure that you are working with good lighting. Good lighting is the amount of light that gives you the best acuity with the least amount of eye strain. Clinical experience has shown that good lighting varies according to the individual; the illumination that is good for one person is not necessarily good for another. It is, however, extremely important that the lighting be optimal for the task you are doing.

Try using natural light as well as light from a lamp or any combination of light arrangements. Don't be afraid to move lamps to different locations—for example, over the shoulder, directly above, or to the side. Watch for glare, however, which can hinder your progress and make you uncomfortable. If you cannot adjust the light to suit your task, let us know so we can design a lighting system that will facilitate your success. Now take a few moments to do the following exercise, which demonstrates the importance of light.

ILLUMINATION EXERCISE

Use the Size and Contrast Reading Materials sheet (opposite page) to experiment with the relationship between the light and the page and your eyes. Start with a 60-watt bulb. If you think you need more light, you may want to move the bulb closer or increase the power of the bulb. First check to make sure the lamp will accept a stronger bulb. Sometimes simple changes—for example, holding the book flat so the full power of the light hits it—can make reading possible.

Notice in this exercise that good lighting lets you read the smaller print in the top half of the page. If you have poorly printed material, however, as in the bottom half of the page, lighting will not help you see the smaller print, even though it is the same size. Using your vision requires contrast, lighting, magnification, proper use of your eyes, and, most important, patience and practice.

3. It is imperative that you not train in a rushed manner. You should do the activities when you are relaxed and happy, not tired or stressed, so you can start and leave your training on a positive note. You should dress comfortably and clear your mind of everything but the task at hand. These learning sessions are no different than practicing to learn a new skill or perfect an old one.

After 15 minutes of home training, you may feel tired or uncomfortable. You may feel as if your eyes are pulling or straining or have a headache or an upset stomach. These are all normal reactions to the initial use of any type of specialized lens system. These feelings should decrease over time, but if they continue or worsen, it is important that you let us know.

4. Sequence of activities for posturing through a near optical system:

a. With the device on or in hand, place the Freeman Near Field Chart at the focal length of the system or at its base, if using a stand magnifier.

Size and Contrast Reading Materials

The size of printed materials
can greatly affect how easily
they can be read, even by people without
visual problems. As you read this text
the print will get smaller and smaller. The
largest print may not be as easy to read as
some of the smaller print, but the smallest print
may be the most difficult to read. Reducing the
amount of light you are reading with can make reading even
more difficult. Try reading this text with good reading light.
Now turn off some of the light and see if it becomes more difficult to read.
You may even find that, with less light, you cannot read as far down this
text as you could with better light. Good reading light is very important for
everyone, but even more important for partially sighted people.

24 point
20 point
18 point
14 point
12 point
10 point
9 point

The quality of print is also very
important in reading. This print
is the same size as the paragraph printed
above, but the contrast has been reduced
by 50%. That is, the print is not as dark,
and it looks gray rather than black. You
will find that it is harder to read this print even in good
lighting than it was to read the previous paragraph, and
it gets even harder as the print gets smaller. Once you read as
much of this paragraph as possible, try reading it again with
some of the lights off. You'll find that you cannot read nearly as well as you could
with better lighting. Good lighting and good reading materials are helpful to
everyone, but may mean the difference between reading and not reading for the partially
sighted person.

24 point
20 point
18 point
14 point
12 point
10 point
9 point

     b. Look through the center of the system and bracket the best position by moving the card toward and away from the system until the best clarity is obtained.

     c. When best clarity through the center of the system is obtained, raise and lower your eyes and repeat the search for best sight.

     5. You have been given the training materials to use while practicing with the new lenses. The only item you need to purchase is a clipboard. Start with single-letter exercises and see how far you can get in 15 minutes. Your progress should improve a little each day. Do not worry if you start to memorize the letters. When the single-letter exercise is so easy that you have no problem seeing and reading it, continue to the exercise with two-letter words. Continue with this sequence until you are comfortable with all of the training sheets. Remember, you can lengthen each of your sessions by an additional 5 minutes if you feel comfortable. It is best, however, not to do this during the first 5 days. It is also wise not to go over 30 minutes during any one session. If you are completing 30-minute sessions comfortably, increasing the number of sessions per day is more productive.

     6. If this activity is difficult because you are trying to look through a blind or blurry spot, eccentric viewing training needs to be added. Call the office and appropriate materials and exercises will be added to your present home training kit.

     7. Visualizing what you want to do is a great way to help you to learn to do an activity better. During the course of the day you may want to visualize what it will be like to successfully hold materials for reading, sewing, playing cards, viewing distance objects through a telescope, and so forth. Following these simple instructions will help you to visualize your activity. You may want to visualize one or two times a day. Here are the steps to follow for visualization:

     a. Find a quiet, dimly lit area.

     b. Sit comfortably with feet flat on the floor, arms uncrossed, and eyes closed, and become aware of your breathing.

c. Start taking deep, slow breaths and say "relax" as you exhale.

d. Concentrate on any tension in your face and around your eyes. Mentally picture this tension like a knot and then visualize this knot becoming undone and limp. You should also feel your face and eye muscles relax. You may also feel your body relax.

e. Tense these same muscles and relax them.

f. Do the same for all your muscles starting with your face and working your way down to your toes—tense first, then relax.

g. Visualize yourself in comfortable surroundings for approximately 2–3 minutes.

h. Mentally begin doing your training, whether it is with a microscope, telescope, hand-held magnifier, or another activity.

i. Feel that you are performing the activity effortlessly.

j. When you finish mentally, put the device down and relax for approximately 30 seconds.

k. Now open your eyes and go about the rest of your day.

Work hard, but enjoy yourself. Call if you have any problems or questions.

Eccentric Viewing I:
16-Point Print with Low Vision Device

You have demonstrated that you are almost ready to begin tracking activities that will help you read print. However, because you cannot use straight-ahead viewing, we have designed materials to help you establish the best off-center viewing spot for you.

SELECTING THE BEST ANGLE FOR ECCENTRIC VIEWING

The following exercises will help you select the best angle for eccentric viewing. Three lines of decreasing thickness appear above each letter or word, and three lines of increasing thickness appear below each letter or word. Starting with the single letters, select the line above or below the letter that allows you to see the letter most clearly; that is, you should center your vision on the line that gives the clearest view of the letter in your peripheral visual field. The following few pages of training materials provide lines of the same height to help you learn eccentric viewing.

E

An

16 pt.

Remember to use your best angle of vision for reading the following materials. Scan each word slowly, saying it aloud. It is more important to use your best viewing angle than it is to read quickly. Your reading speed will improve as you become accustomed to reading this way.

are	key	way
may	the	its
any	see	who

16 pt.

This page is a little more difficult than the last because the words are longer and closer together. Remember, accuracy in using your best viewing angle and in reading each word correctly are still more important than how fast you read.

were	then	seen	ride

list	have	mean	word

with	loud	care	make

fair	open	band	race

16 pt.

This is the last training page. Learning to use your vision is not easy, but it will become easier and you will enjoy reading more.

white   green   black   brown   color

phone   crumb   paste   paint   burnt

while   family   ready   meant   makes

carry   dealt   carve   gravy   great

16 pt.

Eccentric Viewing I:
12-Point Print with Low Vision Device

You have demonstrated that you are almost ready to begin tracking activities that will help you read print. However, because you cannot use straight-ahead viewing, we have designed materials to help establish the best off-center viewing spot for you.

SELECTING THE BEST ANGLE FOR ECCENTRIC VIEWING

The following exercises will help you select the best angle for eccentric viewing. Three lines of decreasing thickness appear above each letter or word, and three lines of increasing thickness appear below each letter or word. Starting with the single letters, select the line above or below the letter that allows you to see the letter most clearly; that is, you should center your vision on the line that gives the clearest view of the letter in your peripheral visual field. The following few pages of training materials provide lines of the same height to help you learn eccentric viewing.

E

An

12 pt.

Use your best angle of vision for reading the following materials. Scan each word slowly, saying it aloud. It is more important to use your best viewing angle than to read quickly. Your reading speed will improve as you become accustomed to reading this way.

are	key	way

may	the	its

any	see	who

12 pt.

This page is a little more difficult than the last because the words are longer and closer together. Accuracy in using your best viewing angle and reading each word correctly are still more important than how fast you read.

were	then	seen	ride

list	have	mean	word

with	loud	care	make

fair	open	band	race

12 pt.

This is the last training page. Learning to use your vision is not easy, but it will become easier and you will enjoy reading more.

white	green	black	brown	color

phone	crumb	paste	paint	burnt

while	family	ready	meant	makes

carry	dealt	carve	gravy	great

12 pt.

Eccentric Viewing I:
8-Point Print with Low Vision Device

You have demonstrated that you are almost ready to begin tracking activities that will help you read print. Because you cannot use straight-ahead viewing, we have designed materials to help you establish the best off-center viewing spot for you.

SELECTING THE BEST ANGLE FOR ECCENTRIC VIEWING

The following exercises will help you select the best angle for eccentric viewing. Three lines of decreasing thickness appear above each letter or word, and three lines of increasing thickness appear below each letter or word. Starting with the single letters, select the line above or below the letter that allows you to see the letter most clearly; that is, you should center your vision on the line that gives the clearest view of the letter in your peripheral visual field. The following few pages of training materials provide lines of the same height to help you practice eccentric viewing.

E

An

8 pt.

Use your best angle of vision when reading the following materials. Scan each word slowly, saying it aloud. It is more important to use your best viewing angle than to read quickly. Your reading speed will improve as you become accustomed to reading this way.

are	key	way
may	the	its
any	see	who

8 pt.

This page is a little more difficult than the last because the words are longer and closer together. Accuracy in using your best viewing angle and in reading each word correctly are still more important than how fast you read.

were	then	seen	ride

list	have	mean	word

with	loud	care	make

fair	open	band	race

8 pt.

This is the last training page. Learning to use your vision is not easy, but it will become easier and you will enjoy reading more.

white	green	black	brown	color

phone	crumb	paste	paint	burnt

while	family	ready	meant	makes

carry	dealt	carve	gravy	great

8 pt.

Eccentric Viewing I:
Eccentric Viewing for Social Situations

The materials required for practicing eccentric viewing in social situations are targets of threshold, superthreshold, and subthreshold sizes.

The target size is determined by converting the distance visual acuity into its components. Targets are divided into three categories according to size: threshold, superthreshold, and subthreshold. For example, if a patient's acuity is 20/200, the threshold target is 3.5 in. tall; a superthreshold target is larger and a subthreshold target is smaller.*

The goal of these exercises is to determine the best prescription for distance viewing to enable the patient to accurately (1) locate a target, (2) identify one target, and (3) grasp a target.

Sequence of Activity

1. Patient is comfortably seated.
2. Have the patient look at your face.
3. Have the patient describe what is visible around your face.
4. Now have the patient look at your shoulders and describe your face.
5. Have the patient alternate between your face and shoulder until the patient is able to best focus on your face.
6. Place targets of varying size around the room.
7. Patient views the first target at superthreshold size 10 ft in front of midline.
8. Patient looks to the left, right, up, and down until target is most clearly identified.
9. Patient looks directly at the target to make it less clear, then to best position of gaze to make it most clear until able to do so accurately.
10. Patient then views other targets and repeats using midline as the reference point.
11. Patient eventually scans from target to target as objects are called out.
12. Repeat the activity at 10, 5, 2.5, and 1 ft. Keep target initially at superthreshold (at readily seen target).
13. When steps 2 through 12 have been successfully completed, repeat while patient is standing.
14. When step 13 has been successfully completed, have the patient walk, stop on command, then repeat viewing.
15. Begin to change target size, first to threshold and repeat steps 6 through 14, then to subthreshold (i.e., a challenging target forcing blur interpretation) and repeat steps 6 through 14.

---

*K Carter. Comprehensive Preliminary Assessment in Low Vision. In R Jose (ed), Understanding Low Vision. New York: AFB Press, 1982.

16. When step 15 has been successfully completed, begin eye-hand activities at near with varying size targets to re-establish a comfortable relationship between the eccentric point of view and reaching. Again, start with superthreshold, eventually ending with subthreshold. The goal of these excersises is to guide smooth eye-hand coordination.

Eccentric Viewing II:
16-Point Print with Low Vision Device

You have demonstrated that you are almost ready to begin tracking activities that will help you read print. However, because you cannot use straight-ahead viewing, we have designed materials to help you establish the best off-center viewing spot for you.

This is designed to help you determine an oblique angle of fixation. The materials have the following form:

$$\overline{}$$

$$\underline{}$$

$$\underline{}$$

123456789

$$\underline{}$$

$$\underline{}$$

$$\underline{}$$

16 pt.

The horizontal angle for fixation is determined in the same way as in Form 5.3a. The oblique angles use the diagonal created by the edges of the three horizontal lines. The top lines are for fixating above objects, and the bottom lines for fixating below objects. The edges on the left can be used for fixating behind the object and the edges on the right can be used for fixating ahead of an object. For reading tasks, it is best to try to move the blind spot superiorly. These fixation skills may be important for activities other than reading.

Selecting the Best Angle for Oblique Eccentric Viewing

The following exercise will help you determine the best angle of viewing. Three lines of decreasing thickness appear above each group of numbers or letters and three lines of increasing thickness appear below them. Starting with the first group of numbers, select the line above or below the numbers that best allows you to see the numbers. The diagonal edges (top left and right and bottom left and right) can be used to determine the best oblique angle. For example, using the middle line below the number centers your eyes on the left edge of the line. What numbers can be seen? Center on the right edge. What numbers can be seen now? One position is usually better than the other, and this is the angle you should practice using. The letters and combinations of letters and numbers on this and subsequent pages can be used to confirm the angle and serve as additional practice materials.

1234567   ABCDEF   1A2B3C4

16 pt.

The following exercises are designed to help you improve your reading ability. Use the reference lines that worked best for you on the previous page. Concentrate on using your vision as accurately as possible and don't worry yet about your reading speed. Increased speed will be gained with the training materials that follow this one. Right now, it is more important to be accurate than fast.

when   zoom   must   bang

seed   even   boot   time

must   fair   cold   heat

16 pt.

Eccentric Viewing II:
12-Point Print with Low Vision Device

You have demonstrated that you are almost ready to begin tracking activities that will help you read print. However, because you cannot use straight-ahead viewing, we have designed materials to help you establish the best off-center viewing spot for you.

This is designed to help you determine an oblique angle of fixation. The materials have the following form:

━━━━━━

───────

──────

123456789

──────

───────

━━━━━━

12 pt.

The horizontal angle for fixation is determined in the same way as in Form 5.3b. The oblique angles use the diagonal created by the edges of the three horizontal lines. The top lines are for fixating above objects, and the bottom lines for fixating below objects. The edges on the left can be used for fixating behind the object to be viewed, while the edges on the right can be used for fixating ahead of an object. For reading tasks it is best to try to move the blind spot superiorly. These fixation skills may be important for activities other than reading.

Keep Practicing

Selecting the Best Angle for Oblique Eccentric Viewing

The following exercise will help you determine the best angle of viewing. Three lines of decreasing thickness appear above each group of numbers or letters and three lines of increasing thickness appear below them. Starting with the first group of numbers, select the line above or below the numbers that best allows you to see the numbers. The diagonal edges (top left and right and bottom left and right) can be used to determine the best oblique angle. For example, using the middle line below the number centers your eyes on the left edge of the line. What numbers can be seen? Center on the right edge. What numbers can be seen now? One position is usually better than the other, and this is the angle you should practice using. The letters and combinations of letters and numbers on this and subsequent pages can be used to confirm the angle and serve as additional practice materials.

1234567	ABCDEF	1A2B3C4

12 pt.

The following exercises are designed to help you improve your reading ability. Use the reference lines that worked best for you on the previous page. Concentrate on using your vision as accurately as possible and do not worry yet about your reading speed. Increased speed will be gained with the training materials that follow this one. Right now, it is more important to be accurate than fast.

when	zoom	must	bang
seed	even	boot	time
must	fair	cold	heat

12 pt.

Eccentric Viewing II:
8-Point Print with Low Vision Device

You have demonstrated that you are almost ready to begin tracking activities that will help you read print. However, because you cannot use straight-ahead viewing, we have designed materials to help you establish the best off-center viewing spot for you.

This is designed to help you determine an oblique angle of fixation. The materials have the following form:

123456789

8 pt.

The horizontal angle for fixation is determined in the same way as in Form 5.3c. The oblique angles use the diagonal created by the edges of the three horizontal lines. The top lines are for fixating above objects and the bottom lines for fixating below objects. The edges on the left can be used for fixating behind the object to be viewed, whereas the edges on the right can be used for fixating ahead of an object. For reading tasks it is best to try to move the blind spot superiorly. These fixation skills may be important for activities other than reading.

Keep Practicing

Selecting the Best Angle for Oblique Eccentric Viewing

The following exercise will help you determine the best angle for viewing. Three lines of decreasing thickness are placed above each group of numbers or letters and three lines of increasing thickness are placed below them. Starting with the first group of numbers, select the line above or below the numbers that best allows you to see the numbers. The diagonal edges (top left and right and bottom left and right) can be used to determine the best oblique angle. For example, using the middle line below the number centers your eyes on the left edge of the line. What numbers can be seen? Center on the right edge. What numbers can be seen now? One position is usually better than the other and this is the angle you should practice using. The letters and combinations of letters and numbers on this and subsequent pages can be used to confirm the angle and serve as additional practice materials.

1234567   ABCDEF   1A2B3C4

8 pt.

The following exercises are designed to help you improve your reading ability. Use the reference lines that worked best for you on the previous page. Concentrate on using your vision as accurately as possible and don't worry yet about your reading speed. Increased speed will be gained with the training materials that follow this one. Right now, it is more important to be accurate than fast.

when	zoom	must	bang

seed	even	boot	time

must	fair	cold	heat

8 pt.

Low Vision
Tracking Exercise—16-Point Print

These tracking sheets are designed to further improve the eye movement skills necessary for reading. The basic sequence begins with single letters followed by two-letter words; three-letter words; four- and five-letter words; six-, seven-, eight-, and nine-letter words; and word columns. When you become proficient with one page, progress to the next page of longer words.

```
W S I M J Z D L T V T D Z M S G I R L X

J Z W O N Q B F S L G X R E F B P H Z F

T P K J S W Z N I W K U T D S B R E E B

P H K N D W Q T Z P J A Y H B M I R A Q

S V T D M T K Z Y V W K W A Y G X M Z Q

I G S O W Y U N K V Q T B P L E R D N Z

F K U J R J G X I Q Z V L P T D N Z O M W

R W U C M E J G X Q I Z V L D E B V P T

R X E M R U Y K N Q B T P Q D R X H Z F

W E X S L U J K L D X Z M J I S W Y N K

G Q O C X L F E R Y A J P N Q M K L T R

W C I M K T L N X R J F I C W A Y H B F S

U C M M I R A X C M Z M E W J W R Z N T
```

Low Vision
Tracking Exercise—16-Point Print

up it in he me on is be no or do go on we

he we am or in we it an if as do of in so

no go on do of or is to we he up it or me

up so go we at am in we he on of so if as

me we is as it am if an we go do up or at

or do up is as he in am at of up go if is

in of up as if an it me in or am we he is

or it up he we on is or to do go on no we

no go do or no be is on as he it in up or

or up do go we an if am it we is he me if

of go no or an do it is me up he or go me

up he go or on is we if he it or do go me

to we as if an in he me am is up or do go

of go up or to am in he as we is me go at

Low Vision
Tracking Exercise—16-Point Print

yes its not let too may saw run men off who

our add red ago had air the any was all yet

and his way got try set six how she has old

out did put top car sea can too use boy you

but dog why end say eat sun for own few far

not run off man say may too try its who yes

yet all was any the air set let got way his

old has she ago six had get red how add our

can you why boy car say sea new cut did out

far few own for sun eat top end use dog but

got way his try six set had she how her has

now red ask any air set the ago men was are

him who its too let man say all not run off

but dog top man sun few yes eat far own end

Low Vision
Tracking Exercise—16-Point Print

well stand want would went ready work house

peace well which show right much green hear

ever under will point such group same happy

until eyes paper when given most south made

said parts even going were north some table

place hand great each clear what thing high

more order head wrong done trees with often

found away train home today door front very

sure horse less times help night days never

woman real those live early here earth does

used funny room might life eerie have apple

think true means read close land three grow

call miles told could page comes left their

money cold black turn young play there last

Low Vision
Tracking Exercise—16-Point Print

animals another within united against

because between making brought places

during country children behind certain

different bigger example writing friend

following second plants however himself

inside important learned cannot looking

across morning saying nothing letters

school picture though perhaps heating

remember letter started several family

something sentences became almost sometimes

through thought turned sentence person

others usually living without together

baseball change working program better

reading wetter states herself brother

newspaper beautiful really outside number

Low Vision
Tracking Exercise—16-Point Print

a	make
and	me
away	my
big	not
blue	one
can	play
come	red
down	run
find	said
for	see
funny	the
go	three
help	to
here	two
I	up
in	we
is	where
it	yellow
jump	you
little	look

Low Vision
Tracking Exercise—16-Point Print

all	out
am	please
are	pretty
at	ran
ate	ride
be	saw
black	say
brown	she
but	so
came	soon
did	that
do	there
eat	they
four	this
get	too
good	under
have	want
he	was
into	well
like	went
must	what
new	white
no	who
now	will
on	with

Low Vision
Tracking Exercise—16-Point Print

about	laugh
better	light
bring	long
carry	much
clean	myself
cut	never
done	only
draw	own
drink	pick
eight	seven
fall	shall
far	show
full	six
got	small
grow	start
hold	ten
hot	today
hurt	together
if	try
keep	warm
kind	most

Low Vision
Tracking Exercise—16-Point Print

always	or
around	pull
because	read
been	right
before	sing
best	sit
both	sleep
buy	tell
call	their
cold	these
does	those
don't	upon
fast	us
first	use
five	very
found	wash
gave	which
goes	why
green	wish
its	work
made	would
many	write
off	your

Low Vision
Tracking Exercise—16-Point Print

from home

I will go

the little children

will look

you are

all night

her father

the red apple

in the garden

what I say

the little chickens

will think

you were

all day

her mother

the red cow

about him

as he said

did not fall

Low Vision
Tracking Exercise—16-Point Print

the yellow ball	to the school	can live
has run away	will walk	it was
he was	on the chair	with us
up there	so long	has made
your mother	the new doll	the black bird
a big horse	could make	by the house
to the house	he would do	if you can
he would try	when you come	can run
the old man	to the barn	from the tree
went away	was made	they are
we are	in the box	at once
down here	to go	will buy
his sister	the funny rabbit	the small boat
some cake	a big house	in the barn
from the farm	when I wish	as I said
as he did	you will like	can fly
the old men	in the grass	to the farm
was found	must be	they were
we were	in the window	at three
up here	to stop	will read
his brother	the funny man	the small boy

Low Vision
Tracking Exercise—12-Point Print

These tracking sheets are designed to further improve the eye movement skills necessary for reading. The basic sequence begins with single letters followed by two-letter words; three-letter words; four- and five-letter words; six-, seven-, eight-, and nine-letter words; and word columns. When you become proficient with one page, progress to the next page.

L D X Z J M I S W Y K N U Q O G A C H F P B R E

T D Z M S N O C W I F J R X L B V E H A G U K Y

N L P K T R O W E J Q Z M C I G S E F B H A V Y

D Z T K W S Q B J F L P C Y N V E R A I M X G O

P I Z M N K T D S V U G Q C O X L F R E H B A Y

C S D T U W V K Y R G O Q N Z M I J A H F B P E

k y u w o s g i c a j m f h z r x e d l p b t v z e r t u

e l h x r a j g f u k y i s c w m o z d n q t p r z l p u

i x g j e c m t r w f o s p t b j y k a l n v d t m n o p

y l c b n j v s e k a w r i t m z q x d h g o u z m p g

s v o q d c x t k l m j z e n r i h p y j n b a w z p t

g o q y v z m w n k j u i a d h s p b c l e x m r e p

r h r f c a g o u k q n y t w s i m z j z x d l t h v r

b y w s i j m z x d l t v p k b r e h a c o g u k f z t

v w k t d y f l b j s c l x e o g x m i r a e v n y z p

h b r f l x c o q t v b p p h a f i j r a v n y y w s g c

c s d j f k y c s m w k y r n b l h p y z r h g o r t z s

4 2 5 3 6 8 9 7 1 3 2 8 5 4 6 3 7 5 9 3 8 5 0 2 1 5

Low Vision
Tracking Exercise—12-Point Print

so an as is do on it if we or in he am is on be up

me an is as at am to if no do it in up or we so go

do of me or so if an we if it or to no as we is he

is up or so in of do as if an it me in or am we he

is if do we is me go to an as up or at am in he as

am if an in he me as is up no to we or do go of he

an is we if he in to me up he go or or do go me in be

to of do it is me up he or go me no at go or no on

at or up do go we as is he me if no of an if am it

no on go up or he do or no be is on we he in it am

me or it up he we on is of or do go on no we it be

so in of do me in or am as if an it we he is up at

go or do up at or up go if is as he in am is do me

if me is he as it am if an we go do up or at me no

it up so go we at am in we he to of so is as or be

we of or is on we no go on do he up it or me in of

is he we if as do of am or in me it an in so go me

we so or up it in he on we is be no or do go no on

Low Vision
Tracking Exercise—12-Point Print

far but why and yes her did add not out few new ago

put six far old air may say eat she any let sea end

its use way any dog try are him you day yes why you

who too she try saw top six use sun was sea the see

say set off old own put one now out new out add red

say far her not cut few has men air car for how ago

any can his eat had may all boy end let are big dog

its and but sea day get him can buy not you and man

put out set use sat may the let sea had its as got

him yet get one new old far own did few see cut for

car sun eat can six top and try big dog why but boy

way add now ago off air run saw any all too are who

yes run saw and its may how eat can our off too who

say own his boy use all any end put old see did boy

men how air car ago few top sun try way you one add

cut let dog way why the its six big are she red not

way day you him are dog use its all six end try not

all may had can any man how for car air eat men but

Low Vision
Tracking Exercise—12-Point Print

ever green eyes group even given each going house

done front door found days does early first down

earth cold every city come could came black close

among book began body best below boys above both

been asked able along away wrong again also after

wind ready will right point high paper hear hard

parts head place home help often have other order

here grow might gave means give never lives good

money feel make smiles face later fire learn fish

light feet large known form kinds from hands food

your small year still half into study idea sound

story know since keep kind short knew shown space

their long these look think line three like last

those land times life today live trees thing less

most using more until make under made which many

would older went stand want place show such happy

same said wrong seen north some clear train sure

horse room woman read seven play funny page apple

Low Vision
Tracking Exercise—12-Point Print

wetter heating baked perhaps toward picture really

nothing number morning states letters enough looking

called learned before important without himself female

however around following turned without should usually

always together living thought father through change

sentence better sometimes others something saying

bought course though started school remember people

glasses letter required family anything several outside

brother newspaper almost beautiful bigger herself friend

became wanted reading second working plants program

mother baseball inside another moving animals become

against cannot because across within between united

things brought answer children making country little

during certain behind different places example around

himself always following better however change writing

father important person learned others looking should

letters turned morning living nothing female picture

almost family became heating course remember perhaps

Low Vision
Tracking Exercise—12-Point Print

a	make
and	me
away	my
big	not
blue	one
can	play
come	red
down	run
find	said
for	see
funny	the
go	three
help	to
here	two
I	up
in	we
is	where
it	yellow
jump	you
little	look

Low Vision
Tracking Exercise—12-Point Print

all	out
am	please
are	pretty
at	ran
ate	ride
be	saw
black	say
brown	she
but	so
came	soon
did	that
do	there
eat	they
four	this
get	too
good	under
have	want
he	was
into	well
like	went
must	what
new	white
no	who
now	will
on	with
our	yes

Low Vision
Tracking Exercise—12-Point Print

about	laugh
better	light
bring	long
carry	much
clean	myself
cut	never
done	only
draw	own
drink	pick
eight	seven
fall	shall
far	show
full	six
got	small
grow	start
hold	ten
hot	today
hurt	together
if	try
keep	warm
kind	most

Low Vision
Tracking Exercise—12-Point Print

always	or
around	pull
because	read
been	right
before	sing
best	sit
both	sleep
buy	tell
call	their
cold	these
does	those
don't	upon
fast	us
first	use
five	very
found	wash
gave	which
goes	why
green	wish
its	work
made	would
many	write
off	your

Low Vision
Tracking Exercise—12-Point Print

from home

I will go

the little children

will look

you are

all night

her father

the red apple

in the garden

what I say

the little chickens

will think

you were

all day

her mother

the red cow

about him

as he said

did not fall

Low Vision
Tracking Exercise—12-Point Print

the yellow ball	to the school	can live
has run away	will walk	it was
he was	on the chair	with us
up there	so long	has made
your mother	the new doll	the black bird
a big horse	could make	by the house
to the house	he would do	if you can
he would try	when you come	can run
the old man	to the barn	from the tree
went away	was made	they are
we are	in the box	at once
down here	to go	will buy
his sister	the funny rabbit	the small boat
some cake	a big house	in the barn
from the farm	when I wish	as I said
as he did	you will like	can fly
the old men	in the grass	to the farm
was found	must be	they were
we were	in the window	at three
up here	to stop	will read
his brother	the funny man	the small boy

Low Vision
Tracking Exercise—8-Point Print

These tracking sheets are designed to further improve the eye movement skills necessary for reading. The basic sequence begins with single letters followed by two-letter words; three-letter words; four- and five-letter words; six-, seven-, eight-, and nine-letter words; and word columns. When you become proficient with one page, progress to the next page.

```
K Q U O G C A H F P B V T D L Z X J I M S Y W N R H W S M

G S B D L X R J F C I W O N O P T D Z V E H A G U K B Q P

W J E X Q I Z G C M S U F B H Y A V D L K N T P R O H Y I

N Y V E A R I M X G O U D H T Z K Q S W B J L F C P D O P

Q O C X F L R B E Y A W J T P N Z K M D T S V U G E R N I

A F H P B S E X F T R Q N Z M J I L M S T D L O R Z T P L E

T L D X Z J M S W N T Y R F H R P B V L E Z I U P B M N R T

a j f z h x r d a l p t b v q n k y u w s o i g m c l m s t z h l c m

c w s o m z n d t q v p b e h x l a r g i g j i r k m n p o q r t w

s p c b l e x f r g o q y n v z w k m u j i t a d h d s g l k e t y l

b s l x r f c w o n q p t d m z s y k g u a e h v k q u d p l m o n

v d t k x n v b r w i t o p w q c r u g r n l p q r s t w v y u o x n

f p u o h g d x z m e t l q r k a w e s w r c f p o z i r c r w r g l

1 9 0 2 3 4 8 5 4 7 5 8 9 1 4 3 7 6 9 4 8 3 2 5 9 7 5 6 7 2 3 4 6

1 5 u y 8 u 0 e 4 5 x 6 v 7 b 8 n 9 m 0 1 s 2 d 3 f 4 g 5 h 6 g 7 j

v d t k m z i p n j w a y h n h b r e f l x c q g u s l g i p r q w m

f p u o h g d x z m t l q r k w a s e v j n b y l f c p o z t r p u m

1 c 8 x 2 9 v 5 i b 3 r 5 o 7 p b 4 5 i v 9 j 6 m 4 r s 6 y p 3 c q

f t b p h k y n a l v d z q i x g j m e c w u r s o c k l r u b v r t y

a j f z h x r d a l w y n y r h k q u o g c a f h r p e b v z d r s l t

i 8 0 3 5 j o 8 6 j 4 p e 3 2 0 j 8 h 9 x 4 2 c v b 5 7 8 h 9 l 8 n j

9 2 8 4 7 5 0 3 1 9 6 0 3 0 6 1 7 4 8 5 3 9 2 6 8 2 4 0 1 8 8 7 4

k 5 h 6 g 0 f 8 d 4 s 1 a 2 q 5 w 0 r 3 t 5 y 7 u 5 p 7 a 3 z 8 p 0
```

Low Vision
Tracking Exercise—8-Point Print

we on no go do or no is on we he in be it up or he am if

go me so in of do as is an it in or am he we is up on at

in me or it up he on is or of do we on go no we in be as

as if so of to he we in am at or we go so up it or no we

be at or up do we an if am it as is he go me if on an up

do is if go or at am in he up as is up do or go if in of

am up is he we or in me it an if as do of in so go be it

it we no go do of or is on we up it or me in as so he

he or up in it he we on is be no or do go he no on we is at

or if me he is as it am if an we go he do up or at be in

am no me go or he up me is it do on or no go of to it we

in me go do or it he we is an or go he up me is an or if

no to go do or up is as me he in an if am we to go is be

me is we of to go as he am at or up do if is go in on do

up is he we am or in me it an if as of in so at go to do

to or it he we as if an we is me if so or do of on be is

so we up in is an me it do no of to am or at or as he up

is am in or up be we it if on he do is at an so in go he

or at be do up we if am it an is me he go if or as me no

am up it or go so at we in he we of to if so or as be do

we on no go or do be no is on we he it in up or he at is

go no to am if an in he me as is up or we do go of in be

in so an at is do it if we up be or in he on am is on we

Low Vision
Tracking Exercise—8-Point Print

day why dog top end for eat sun few own yes far but out

use new put did cut say sea car can you big boy our now

red get ago six had she how her has old his and got add

way set the air was any are all yet you boy use big try

sea can say car did put new out yes him who its too cut

let say man run may not off for yes far few own had saw

eat sun end top why day but off not run men may saw dog

man let too its who him yet are was all ago the set yes

air any ask red now our has her how she had six got old

try his way get and day but why end top eat sun for dog

own far few yes new out did put say car sea can use cut

boy now our add you red ago get had six how she has big

old her and his way got try set the any was all yet air

are him yes its who let too may saw run men off not man

big yes far few own for sun eat top end why dog but day

use did can you say car boy sea cut her out put old new

has she how all six try had got way his and get are yet

was any the air set ago red add run our now not off men

cut man saw may too let who its yes put him new out did

say car sea can use big boy day dog why you but and too

eat sun for own few far not off men man run may yes

yes was too set let air who the its any saw him all are yet

try way get had his six and how ago got her she old has

Low Vision
Tracking Exercise—8-Point Print

also about from heard half must water side after wind small

your still year words away again find kinds into sound hands

more soon along able known from study idea write mean where

asked that been story food while just above name light large

they since back fast among know learn next space this world

white both below four keep short need whole them later began

boys lives five kind years near being shown then makes best

there face young knew over money time their black body comes

fish like miles only these than funny could book class feel

means think once apple take every came long might fire three

line look seven open earth tell never come those good woman

horse early part night took times city give first last order

page today turn often train cold found gave left trees play

wrong told front call other grow land clear thing read great

true north place down table have life going room parts used

south does using here live paper rest until given upon happy

days going help older point less under sure very green door

right home which many seen house with peace read done would

head stand more water small what heard each about hand said

words make were still some after where even sound high kinds

made again same write when eyes known hard along study most

while such story will ever asked hear world much since large

show light work above ways will white went space want learn

Low Vision
Tracking Exercise—8-Point Print

making places herself things beautiful brother united

outside within moving anything across newspaper required

become glasses cannot inside started mother several remember

wanted plants sentences second something through friend

sentence bigger thought sometimes almost became together

course usually family without following letter people

school himself though important bought learned however

saying looking always change morning better letters nothing

father living perhaps others heating should another picture

animals person against turned female because around between

before brought called enough country children looked certain

different really example toward writing states number

saying heating wetter glasses moving without bigger perhaps

example required better usually within female picture

friend person different bought anything together states

newspaper noting united certain wanted though between

turned letters toward things beautiful second children

school sentence looking should brought really sometimes

places herself plants people thought others learned brother

number something important mother because making letter

reading living sentences himself little working looked

program inside several family however father against enough

Low Vision
Tracking Exercise—8-Point Print

a	make
and	me
away	my
big	not
blue	one
can	play
come	red
down	run
find	said
for	see
funny	the
go	three
help	to
here	two
I	up
in	we
is	where
it	yellow
jump	you
little	look

Low Vision
Tracking Exercise—8-Point Print

about	laugh
better	light
bring	long
carry	much
clean	myself
cut	never
done	only
draw	own
drink	pick
eight	seven
tall	shall
far	show
full	six
got	small
grow	start
hold	ten
hot	today
hurt	together
if	try
keep	warm
kind	most

Low Vision
Tracking Exercise—8-Point Print

always	or
around	pull
because	read
been	right
before	sing
best	sit
both	sleep
buy	tell
call	their
cold	these
does	those
don't	upon
fast	us
first	use
five	very
found	wash
gave	which
goes	why
green	wish
its	work
made	would
many	write
off	your

Low Vision
Tracking Exercise—8-Point Print

from home

I will go

the little children

will look

you are

all night

her father

the red apple

in the garden

what I say

the little chickens

will think

you were

all day

her mother

the red cow

about him

as he said

did not fall

Low Vision
Tracking Exercise—8-Point Print

the yellow ball	to the school	can live
has run away	will walk	it was
he was	on the chair	with us
up there	so long	has made
your mother	the new doll	the black bird
a big horse	could make	by the house
to the house	he would do	if you can
he would try	when you come	can run
the old man	to the barn	from the tree
went away	was made	they are
we are	in the box	at once
down here	to go	will buy
his sister	the funny rabbit	the small boat
some cake	a big house	in the barn
from the farm	when I wish	as I said
as he did	you will like	can fly
the old men	in the grass	to the farm
was found	must be	they were
we were	in the window	at three
up here	to stop	will read
his brother	the funny man	the small boy

Proficiency Activities—Near

MICROSCOPIC WORD SEARCH

Materials: A microscope of appropriate power, word search activity of appropriate size, a stopwatch or watch with a second hand. Your doctor will provide some of the materials.

Goals: To efficiently use the microscope to see and sequence information.

To be able to use a pencil, pen, or marker while viewing through the microscope.

To reinforce visual tracking and visual memory.

Sequence of Activity:

1. Place the word search paper on a clipboard at the appropriate distance from the microscope.

2. View the word to be found.

3. Sequentially track the information in the word search puzzle from left to right and line by line using the full field of the microscope to view letters to left, right, above, below, and diagonal from the fixated letter.

4. When you believe a word has been found, mark the spot and sequentially track the letters until verification has been made.

5. When this is accomplished with relative ease, do the activity under timed conditions to increase automaticity of movement.

6. When successful, increase the difficulty of the word search (i.e., more words).

MICROSCOPIC TRACKING

Materials: A microscope of appropriate power, reading pages of appropriate size in this book, a Michigan tracking series of appropriate size (available from Bernell Corporation, South Bend, IN; see below), a stopwatch or a watch with a second hand. Your doctor will provide some of these materials.

Goal: To use the microscopic lens smoothly and efficiently.

Sequence of Activity:

1. Put the microscope on and bring the material to the focal length of the system (point of sharpest image).
2. Hold the material parallel to the face. Use a clipboard for stability if necessary.
3. Call out letters, numbers, or words in sequence under untimed conditions.
4. Once you are comfortable, time yourself as a challenge to increase your skill level.

a b c d e f g h i j k l m n o p q r s t u v w x y z

Foth nar bolhy melk roce toreup. Ix
shir dop tulf ursh mil pherk zoth.
Lofit rikk lun raug muiq thau quat
urlk yat duils. Veem ebn jop tarud
thec fobt klab non mer. Zurt derub
ird. Chen ferv yath gorf tach taipe
geuba dequi reet skug falm cheab.
Phed telc dawl dumn wenk voip maf
mewp nals norf. Mex opj denoy zaab

_____ Min. _____ Sec.

WRITING FROM A MICROSCOPIC POSTURE

Materials: Paper with bold or heavy raised lines, pen or pencil, marker, list of words, microscope, ruler, typoscope.

Goal: To be able to write with a microscopic lens confidently.

Sequence of Activity:

1. Take a pen, pencil, or marker and sit comfortably at a table.

2. Place lined, raised lined, or unlined paper at the appropriate writing angle and distance. You may need a ruler or typoscope to feel more confident drawing in a straight line.

3. Place the pen, pencil, or marker on the page in the upper left corner of the page.

4. Close your eyes and sit in a natural writing posture.

5. When words are called out, write them down using your muscle memory.

6. Verify the word visually using your microscope.

7. Once you have completed steps 1 through 6 successfully, assume a posture consistent with the work distance of your microscope but do not wear the microscope.

8. When the list of words is repeated, write the words at this new distance with your eyes closed.

9. Verify the word using the microscope.

10. Repeat steps 7 and 8 with the microscope, with your eyes open.

MONOVISION

Materials: A microscopic lens, patch, Hart chart (available from Bernell Corporation; see next page). Your doctor will provide these materials.

Goal: To allow you to view both distance and near using a microscopic lens in front of one eye and a clear lens or distance prescription in front of the other eye.

Sequence of Activity:

1. With the nonreading eye occluded, hold the materials at the appropriate focal length of your microscope and follow the standard training procedures to encourage proper use of the microscope.

2. Once you are comfortably reading with the microscope, the occluded eye should be unoccluded. You should attempt to open that eye while reading with the microscope or doing another near activity.

3. If binocular vision interferes with use of the microscope, the eye should be closed again (preferably by you) or occluded with a filter or patch.

4. Continue training until success has been achieved and you can read with both eyes open. Your doctor will give you activities that require near/far viewing. These should first be done while seated. One activity may be Hart chart activities with the near chart held at the focal length of the lens and the distance chart held at 10–12 ft with print size commensurate with your measured distance visual acuities. Another activity may involve the use of other reading material or television viewing. These activities should be done with the material in front of you.

5. Once step 4 has been performed successfully, steps 1 through 4 should be repeated while standing.

6. Once step 5 has been comfortably accomplished, scan the room at distance and, from time to time, pick up the Hart chart reading material, read, and then scan the room again.

7. Once step 6 is performed in a stationary position, you should walk slowly in a familiar environment with a guide. There should be no steps or rises in the selected environment. The assistant should encourage you to periodically stop, scan the room, pick up something to read, put the reading material down, and continue to scan the room.

8. Once you have achieved comfort in familiar territory, you can then attempt to explore unfamiliar territory. This must be done with a guide.

It is important throughout this entire activity that scanning be done with the unoccluded distance eye, especially to learn to scan the side to which the microscopic lens has been fitted.

	2		4		6		8		10
1	O	F	N	P	V	D	T	C	H	E
	Y	B	A	K	O	E	Z	L	R	X
3	E	T	H	W	F	M	B	K	A	P
	B	X	F	R	T	O	S	M	V	C
5	R	A	D	V	S	X	P	E	T	O
	M	P	O	E	A	N	C	B	K	F
7	C	R	G	D	B	K	E	P	M	A
	F	X	P	S	M	A	R	D	L	G
9	T	M	U	A	X	S	O	G	P	B
	H	O	S	N	C	T	K	U	Z	L

Form 5.6 *(continued)*

HAND MAGNIFICATION USE WITH CONVENTIONAL BIFOCAL GLASSES

Materials: A hand-held magnifier, tape, your bifocal prescription.

Goal: To achieve maximum magnification and field of view with a hand-held magnifier.

Sequence of Activity:

1. Your bifocal will be taped so that it is frosted.

2. Place the hand-held magnifier on printed material of appropriate size.

   a. Place the printed material at a comfortable working distance on a horizontal or slightly angled surface (e.g., lap desk or table).

   OR

   b. Tape the printed material on a wall at a comfortable working distance.

3. While looking through the distance portion of the lens, slowly lift the hand-held magnifier from the page until the print clears and then blurs.

4. Move the magnifier closer to and away from the page to find the best viewing distance and the greatest magnification.

5. When step 4 is achieved automatically, remove the tape. You can also demonstrate how the hand-held magnifier can be modified by doing the following:

   a. Repeat steps 2 and 4 while viewing through the bifocal.

   b. Verify a change in magnification.

   c. Discuss the advantages for using the hand-held magnifier at full magnification and less magnification with your doctor.

6. Grasp the viewing material in one hand and the hand magnifier in the other hand and repeat steps 3 and 4. Practice moving the hand-held magnifier and viewing material to various distances.

FIXED-FOCUS STAND MAGNIFIER USE WITH NEAR PRESCRIPTION

Materials: A stand magnifier, tape, your reading prescription or bifocal.

Goal: To achieve maximum magnification and field of view with a fixed-focus stand magnifier with diverging rays.

Sequence of Activity:

1. Tape the distance part of your prescription so that only the bifocal is usable. The doctor may do this for you.

2. Place the stand magnifier on the viewing material.

3. Bring the stand magnifier/viewing material combination slowly toward the bifocal until maximum clarity is achieved. Move the magnifier/material back and forth to obtain the position that gives you the best magnification and clarity.

4. Once you are successful with this activity, remove the tape from the distance part of the prescription and repeat the activity.

Low Vision Homework Instructional Materials—Distance

You have been shown various techniques for the efficient use of telescopic systems in our office. Now it is up to you to practice these skills at home. Before starting the activities consider these hints:

1. You should work on your home activities for no longer than 15 minutes at a time. Fifteen minutes seems to be the appropriate amount of time one can initially work without becoming frustrated or uncomfortable. These 15-minute work sessions should be done three times a day, 5 days a week. As you work, if you find that 15 minutes goes by quickly and you are not having any problems, increase your time by 5-minute intervals. It is best, however, not to do this during the first 5 days. It is also wise not to work more than 30 minutes during one session. If you are completing 30-minute sessions comfortably, increasing the number of sessions per day is more productive.

2. During the 15-minute session, ensure that you are working with good lighting. Good lighting is the amount of light that gives you the best acuity with the least amount of eye strain. Clinical experience has shown that good lighting varies according to the individual; the illumination that is good for one person is not necessarily good for another. It is, however, extremely important that the lighting be optimal for the task you are doing. Once you go outside, however, lighting will be difficult to control. Therefore, practice inside with good light until you are comfortable enough to enter an environment in which you will be unable to control the lighting.

3. It is imperative that you not train in a rushed manner. You should do it when you are relaxed and happy, not tired or stressed. That way you can start and leave your training on a positive note. You should be dressed comfortably and your mind should be cleared of everything but the task at hand. These learning sessions are no different than practicing to learn a new skill or perfect an old one.

4. Telescopic work can be extremely frustrating because, unlike working at near, you do not have control over what you are viewing. In an effort to minimize frustration, you may want to follow this sequence of activities. Remember, these are guidelines. You will find that after a while you will develop your own strategy.

a. Locate a stationary object with your eye. Stand 15–20 feet from the object. If you have a hand-held telescope, lift it to your eye. If you have a head-borne system, lower your head while raising your eye so that you can look through the telescope.

Focus the telescope on the target. Once the target is clear, identify as much detail as you can and the amount of area you see. Now put the telescope down and move 5 feet closer to the target. Refocus and repeat the previous step of identifying detail and field. Repeat this until you are as close as you can get to the target until focusing will no longer clarify the image. Now, reverse the process.

b. Position yourself about 20 feet away from a group of separated objects to be viewed. Locate the objects first with your eye and then through the telescope. If you have a hand-held device, practice raising the telescope to your eye, viewing the targets by looking through the telescope and moving your head, then lowering the telescope. Your goal should be to move quickly and efficiently, lifting the telescope to your eye, then locating, identifying, and putting the telescope back down. If you are using a head-borne device, the same concept applies. Locate the target, look through the telescope, identify the targets, and then move your eye out of the telescope. Once you are able to do this smoothly and efficiently with your hand-held or head-borne telescope, change distances, refocus, and repeat the procedure.

c. When stationary objects become easy to see, locate a moving target, (e.g., a person or vehicle) while you are stationary. Track the target with your unaided vision, lock in on the target, and, if your telescope is hand-held, lift it to your eye and track the object. With a head-borne telescope, lower your head so your eye moves into the telescope and follow the target.

   d. Now that you have gotten this far, you may want to use the same principles to track a stationary object while moving.

   Remember these points:

- Once the telescope is up to your eye, objects are going to move more quickly than normal.

- Targets will move in a direction opposite the movement of the telescope. If you scan to the left, the targets will move quickly to the right. This is called *movement parallax* or *speed smear* and may initially make you uncomfortable.

- Moving targets are significantly more difficult to work with than stationary targets regardless of whether they are moving or you are moving.

- If you are using a monocular system, you might initially want to close the eye that you are not using. Over time, however, having both eyes open will be more efficient.

- In any activity you do with your telescope, be sure to use the telescope in a logical and sequential scanning pattern. If a target is difficult to see with the telescope, first locate the area you want to view, find a more obvious object around the target, bring the telescope to your eye, locate that object, then sequentially scan the area until you are able to locate and identify what you wish to see.

   e. Once you can do these activities easily, try to enhance your visual memory skills by looking through your telescope, identifying a scene, then closing your eyes and attempting to remember everything you have seen through the telescope. This will help increase your ability to get as much information as you can as efficiently as possible.

   Your success in using a telescope depends greatly upon your motivation and efficiency. As you use your telescope more often in your environment, your skill level will improve. Recognize that although the telescope may not be as cosmetically appealing as a designer frame, you will perform significantly better using this device. As in any other segment of training, if you have any problems please feel free to call us.

After 15 minutes of home training, you may feel tired or uncomfortable or feel like your eyes are pulling or straining. You may have a headache or an upset stomach. These are all normal reactions to the initial use of any type of unconventional lens system. These feelings should decrease over time, but if they continue or worsen, it is important that you let us know.

5. Visualizing what you want to do is a great way to help you to learn to do an activity better. During the course of the day you may want to visualize what it will be like to successfully hold materials for reading, sewing, playing cards, viewing distance objects through a telescope, and so forth. Following these simple instructions will help you to visualize your activity. You may want to visualize one or two times a day. Here are the steps for visualizing:

a. Find a quiet, dimly lit area.

b. Sit comfortably with feet flat on the floor, arms uncrossed, and eyes closed, and become aware of your breathing.

c. Start taking deep, slow breaths and say "relax" as you exhale.

d. Concentrate on any tension in your face and around your eyes. Mentally picture this tension like a knot and then visualize this knot becoming undone and limp. You should also feel your face and eye muscles relax. You may also feel your body relax.

e. Tense these same muscles and relax them.

f. Do the same for all your muscles starting with your face and working your way down to your toes—tense first, then relax.

g. Visualize yourself in comfortable surroundings for approximately 2–3 minutes.

h. Mentally begin doing your training, whether it is with a microscope, telescope, hand-held magnifier, or another activity.

i. Feel that you are performing the activity effortlessly.

j. When you finish mentally, put the device down and relax for approximately 30 seconds.

k. Now open your eyes and go about the rest of your day.

Work hard, but enjoy yourself. Call if you have any problems or questions.

Proficiency Activities—Distance

COLE TECHNIQUE* FOR HOLDING A HAND TELESCOPE

Materials: A hand-held telescope, various targets. The telescope and some targets may be provided by your doctor.

Goal: To view through a hand-held telescope with minimal effort.

Sequence of Activity:

1. Focus your telescope for 10 feet.

2. Hold your telescope in the dominant hand with a palmar grasp (i.e., grasping it with the palm of your hand, your fingers and thumb wrapped around the telescope).

3. Bring the hand with the telescope to your eye, and stabilize the telescope by resting the joint and lower half of the thumb on the side of your nose.

4. Hold the eyepiece lens of the telescope as close as possible to your eye while looking through the telescope. You should be looking through a complete circle. If not, move the telescope until your eye is centered in the eyepiece lens and you see a circle of vision.

5. View a large target directly in front of you.

6. When this is successful, track that target or another moving target at the same distance.

7. Decrease the size of target to as small an object as you can identify through the telescope.

8. Repeat steps 4 and 5.

9. Increase the distance for the target.

10. Focus the telescope with the free hand and repeat steps 5 through 7.

---

*Developed by Dr. Roy Cole, State University of New York, College of Optometry.

TELESCOPE FIELD AWARENESS

Materials: A hand-held or spectacle-mounted telescope, chalkboard or other vertical writing surface, chalk, pen.

Goal: To give you an appreciation of the functional field of view of your prescribed telescope.

This should be done in the office first and then repeated at home.

Sequence of Activity:

1. Place an X of appropriate size on a chalkboard or writing surface (e.g., paper taped to the wall). Begin with an **X** larger than necessary for you to see.

2. Stand 10 feet from the chalkboard and view the **X** through the telescope. The telescope should be as close to your eye as possible. The other eye should be occluded.

3. Have someone bring a visible target from outside the viewing area of the telescope until it is seen in the periphery of the telescope. Mark this position on the chalkboard. Repeat this from the right, left, up, and down until the area of vision through the telescope is drawn on the chalkboard. This area represents your functional field of view with the telescope.

4. Repeat at 20, 5, and 2.5 feet. What happens to the functional field of view?

5. Repeat with the telescope 1, 2, and 3 inches away from your eye. What happens to the functional field of view?

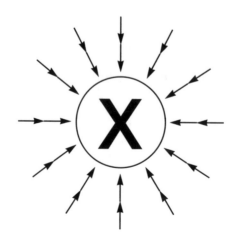

PERCEPTUAL CONCEPTS THROUGH A TELESCOPE

Materials: A hand-held or spectacle-mounted telescope of appropriate power and any scene that can be viewed with a telescope.

Goal: To look through a telescope and describe what you see both through the telescope and outside the viewing area of the telescope.

Your doctor will demonstrate this in the clinic.

Sequence of Activity:

1. Place the hand-held or spectacle-mounted telescope in front of the eye.

2. Once the telescope is focused on a target, describe the target and what is surrounding the target (outside the telescope—not magnified), as best you can.

3. Scan the whole scene with the telescope to determine whether you were accurate in your description.

4. Put the telescope down. Identify as much information about the scene as you can remember.

TELESCOPIC PURSUIT AND TRACKING ACTIVITIES

Materials: A hand-held or spectacle-mounted telescope of appropriate power, rotator, and Hart charts.

Goal: To learn to use the telescope to track efficiently with speed and accuracy.

This is an in-office activity.

Sequence of Activity:

1. Sit approximately 10 feet from the rotator with a Hart chart on it.
2. View the Hart chart and call out letters after focusing the telescope for that distance.
3. When successful, move the rotator clockwise. Call out letters again.
4. Step 3 should be repeated with the chart rotating counter-clockwise.
5. When steps 3 and 4 have been successfully completed, the activity should be repeated at 5 feet, 2.5 feet, and at the closest focal point of the telescope.

TELESCOPIC CONTROLLED READER

Materials: A hand-held or spectacle-mounted telescope of appropriate power, a controlled reader, and appropriately sized materials.

Goal: To teach you to use the telescope with speed and accuracy.

This is an in-office activity.

Sequence of Activity:

1. Sit 10 feet from the screen.
2. The controlled reader is set for speed and/or movement, based on your capabilities.
3. Say aloud what is seen. Begin with sequences of one to two letters, numbers, or symbols.
4. As you progress, the speed or movement of the controlled reader is increased, and the sequence of letters, numbers, and symbols increases.

Form 5.8 *(continued)*

TELESCOPIC TRACKING

Materials: A telescope, chalkboard, vertical writing surface, chalk, pen, and marker.

Goal: To teach you to use the telescope efficiently for systematic tracking, localization, and tracing.

This will be demonstrated in the office first and then repeated at home.

Sequence of Activity:

1. Place a series of numbers or letters or a combination on a surface in a repeating pattern. Connect the characters with arrows as shown in Diagram A.

2. With the telescope, follow the path (from left to right), calling out each character.

3. This should be performed at 10, 5, 2.5, and 1 foot.

4. Repeat steps 1 through 3 without the lines between the characters, as shown in Diagram B.

5. When you have successfully completed steps 1 through 4, randomly place characters on a surface and locate specific characters in sequence using systematic scanning. Diagram C demonstrates the task of finding the numbers 1 through 24 in sequence.

6. This should be performed at 10, 5, 2.5, and 1 foot.

A

1	6	7	B	u
3	2	x	y	7
c	8	g	z	10
13	3	d	h	i
4	19	e	15	j
0	s	e	3	13

B

1	6	7	B	u
3	2	x	y	7
c	8	g	z	10
13	3	d	h	i
4	19	e	15	j
0	s	e	3	13

C

1	17	3	7	18
12	4	10	2	5
6	16	2	11	19
20	23	22	24	21
15	9	14	8	13

TELESCOPIC TACHISTOSCOPIC ACTIVITY

Materials: A hand-held or spectacle-mounted telescope, chalkboard, flip chart, and an 8 × 11 sheet of paper or cardboard with a large **X** on it.

Goal: To enhance visual confidence with short-term viewing through a telescope.

This is an in-office exercise. It can be repeated at home.

Sequence of Activity:

1. Focus the telescope for 10 feet.
2. Have an assistant tape a character on the chalkboard or flip chart at the 10-foot viewing distance.
3. The assistant should cover the character with the 8 × 11 sheet of paper.
4. Pick up the focused telescope and view the **X** on the 8 × 11 sheet of paper.
5. The assistant says, "Ready—Now." On the "Now" command, the assistant removes the 8 × 11 sheet of paper, allowing you to view the target for a specific period of time before covering the target again. (Allotted time should be 1 second per character.)
6. You are to identify the character when the paper is removed. If you cannot identify the character in this amount of time, allow additional seconds until you become proficient in this task.
7. Once you are successful, increase the number of characters and repeat steps 3 through 6.
8. Repeat steps 1 through 7 at 1, 2.5, 5, and 20 feet. When this is accomplished with minimal difficulty, proceed to step 9.
9. View the 8 × 11 sheet of paper with the **X** at 10 feet without the telescope. The **X** may be blurry, but look where the blur is.
10. On the command "Ready," put the telescope to your eye and view the **X** through it.

11. On the command "Now," the target is uncovered for a specified period of time for you to try to identify.

12. Once the target is covered, again call out the sequence of characters.

13. Decrease the amount of time the characters are viewed.

14. Decrease the time between the commands "Ready" and "Now."

15. Repeat steps 9 through 14 at 1, 2.5, 5, and 20 feet.

TELESCOPE ADAPTATION

Materials: A hand-held or spectacle-mounted telescope and multiple targets.

Goal: For you to appreciate changes in environmental lighting and respond accordingly.

Sequence of Activity:

1. Place the focused telescope to the eye.
2. At 10 feet, view a detailed target; identify all its important points and critical detail.
3. Decrease the lighting, adjust to the change, and refixate on another target.
4. Repeat under various lighting conditions with differing distances and various sized targets. (All targets must be detailed—e.g., clocks, photographs, drawings, posters, calendars.)

Form 5.8 *(continued)*

TELESCOPE PERIPHERAL AWARENESS ACTIVITY

Materials: A spectacle-mounted telescope, buntball and bat, and target.
Goal: To make the patient aware of peripheral information while viewing centrally through a telescope to enable simultaneous processing.

This activity must be supervised in the office setting.

Sequence of Activity:

1. Have the patient identify the field of view through the telescope. Have the patient modify vertex distance to maximize the field of view based on position.
2. Have the patient view a target through a telescope (e.g., Hart chart, Designs for Vision Chart). Have the patient identify characters through the telescope. While looking through the telescope, the patient should tell you what is being seen peripherally.
3. With no correction, have the patient take a bat and hit a buntball while viewing it directly. The ball should be big enough to be seen but not necessarily clearly. Try to get the patient to be in control of the movement of the ball while viewing directly. Then have the patient repeat the same activity while looking ahead and viewing the target peripherally.
4. Combine telescopic viewing with peripheral awareness. While viewing through the telescope, have the patient bunt a large ball placed at waist level.
5. When step 4 can be done with minimal difficulty, call out positions on the bat to be used, for example, left, right, and so forth.

Low Vision Homework
Instructional Materials—Peripheral

You have been shown some techniques for the efficient use of your peripheral vision in our office. Now it is up to you to begin to learn these skills at home. Before starting these activities, consider these hints:

1. Your home activities should initially be done for no longer than 15 minutes at a time.

2. When doing these activities, you should always make sure that someone is with you to maintain safety.

3. Begin any activity in a familiar environment and with a relaxed manner. Do not attempt any activity while you are stressed or tired. This way you can start and leave your training on a positive note.

4. You should be dressed comfortably and your mind should be clear of everything but the task at hand. These learning sessions are no different than practicing to learn a new skill or perfect an old one.

5. Visualizing what you want to do is a great way to help you to learn to do an activity better. During the course of the day you may want to visualize what it will be like to successfully hold materials for reading, sewing, playing cards, viewing distance objects through a telescope, and so forth. Following these simple instructions will help you to visualize your activity. You may want to visualize one or two times a day. Here are the steps for visualizing:

   a. Find a quiet, dimly lit area.

   b. Sit comfortably with feet flat on the floor, arms uncrossed, and eyes closed, and become aware of your breathing.

   c. Start taking deep, slow breaths and say "relax" as you exhale.

   d. Concentrate on any tension in your face and around your eyes. Mentally picture this tension like a knot and then visualize this knot becoming undone and limp. You should also feel your face and eye muscles relax. You may also feel your body relax.

e. Tense these same muscles and relax them.

f. Do the same for all your muscles starting with your face and working your way down to your toes—tense first, then relax.

g. Visualize yourself in comfortable surroundings for approximately 2–3 minutes.

h. Mentally begin doing your training, whether it is with a microscope, telescope, hand-held magnifier, or another activity.

i. Feel that you are performing the activity effortlessly.

j. When you finish mentally, put the device down and relax for approximately 30 seconds.

k. Now open your eyes and go about the rest of your day.

Work hard, but enjoy yourself. Call if you have any problems or questions.

Proficiency Activities—Peripheral

PERIPHERAL AWARENESS TRAINING WITH A PRISM

Material: A prism.

Goal: To teach the patient how to look into a prism and become aware of targets in the periphery on the side of the field loss.

This activity is best done in the office under supervision.

Sequence of Activity:

1. Place the prism base out on the field-loss side (10–30Δ is recommended). The apex of the prism should be approximately 2 mm from the patient's cardinal position of gaze so that the edge of the prism is not noticed with both eyes open.

2. With the patient seated, a discussion of the use of the prism should proceed as follows: "You are to look into the prism every 8–10 seconds just as you would look into the rear view mirror of a car, actively appreciating what is on the side where the field loss has occurred."

3. Having given this information, the practitioner should sit opposite the patient. On the field-loss side, the practitioner will hold up a different number of fingers every 8–10 seconds. When the patient looks into the prism, the fingers should be counted. The practitioner should change the numbers and the position of the hand as the patient resumes looking straight ahead.

   When this is done comfortably and efficiently in a seated position, tell the patient to stand and repeat this.

4. When step 3 is done comfortably and efficiently while standing, tell the patient to walk slowly in a safe environment with minimal obstructions, repeating the same activity.

5. When step 4 is performed comfortably and efficiently, encourage the patient to go with a partner to an enclosed environment such as a mall and perform the same activity. The partner should walk on the patient's full-field side. (The partner should always be visually aware of the patient's field-loss side so the partner can intercede in the event of a potential accident.) During the course of this training, the patient should tell the partner everything that is being seen and try to predict movement on the field-loss side.

6. When step 5 is performed comfortably and efficiently, encourage the patient to move into other environments, some familiar and some unfamiliar, and repeat the same process until the patient is fully comfortable with his or her awareness on that side.

PERIPHERAL AWARENESS TRAINING WITH A HANGING BALL

Materials: A hanging ball and a prism.

Goal: To teach the patient awareness of field loss.

This is best accomplished in the office.

Sequence of Activity:

1. The patient is seated.
2. The hanging ball is moved on the sighted side. A hanging ball can be any size or color. It is typically hung from the ceiling.
3. The patient attempts to locate the hanging ball on command.
4. The hanging ball is moved to the blind side.
5. The patient attempts to locate the hanging ball on command by
   a. Turning the head
   b. Viewing into the prism
6. Repeat steps 2 through 5 with the patient standing.
7. Repeat steps 2 through 5 with the patient walking.

PRISM BALANCE

Materials: Balance board, walk rail, and prism.
Goal: To teach the patient to maintain balance with field loss.
This activity must be conducted in the office.
Sequence of Activity:

1. The patient is to balance on the balance board without using the prism.
   a. The patient's feet should be shoulder-width apart.
   b. The patient should fixate on a target 10 ft away. Balance should be attempted from the waist down using hip and knee flexion/extension only. Once successful, the patient should view targets to either side of fixation using separation of variable distances. Once peripheral to central localization is accomplished, proceed to step 2.
2. The patient is to balance on the balance board with prism on (prism should have been set appropriately on lens carrier). Setting is appropriate when the patient has no awareness of the prism when viewing straight ahead in primary gaze and only has to move the eyes minimally to view through the prism. The prism is to be affixed base out to the lens carrier and monocularly on the side of the field loss.
3. The patient is to walk on the walk rail without the prism.
4. The patient is to walk on the walk rail with the prism on and scan to the side of field loss, calling out what is seen.

MIRROR FIXATIONS FOR FIELD LOSS

Material: A hand or spectacle-mounted mirror.

Goal: To make you aware of the field loss and/or neglected area.

This activity should be demonstrated in the office first and repeated at home.

Sequence of Activity:

1. Identify the area of field loss.
2. With a hand mirror, while seated, place the mirror above the eye on the sighted-field side.
3. Look into the mirror to appreciate information in the unsighted field. This information is reversed as in any mirror system.
4. The mirror is then used as a scanning mechanism by rotating it around a vertical axis for awareness of information in the area of field loss.
5. Once this is done successfully, stand and repeat steps 1 through 4 until they can be performed automatically.
6. Once step 5 is performed with confidence, move about in a familiar environment (e.g., at home), periodically pick up the mirror, scan as in steps 2 through 5, and then place the mirror down while continuing to move.
7. Once step 6 is performed, go to unfamiliar environments with a partner and repeat step 6. Talk about all the information seen in the mirror. Always be visually alert while this activity is being performed.

FIELD AWARENESS FOR HEMIANOPIC OR FIELD-NEGLECT PATIENTS

Materials: Strings and beads.

Goal: To train the hemianopic or field-neglect patient to appreciate information in the field loss or neglected field area.

This must be performed in the office under supervision.

Sequence of Activity:

1. Tie a series of strings to a number of objects in the training area on what appears to be the blind side for the patient.
2. If necessary, color code the string to help the patient see and differentiate each string and conceptualize what is to be looked at by color.
3. Have the patient sit facing the work area so that the patient's midline bisects the field of activity.
4. Have the patient pick a string up with the hand on the field-awareness side.
5. Have the patient tighten the string and then visually follow the string to the anchored object. If this is too difficult, put a bead on the string, and have the patient follow the bead visually while it is moved from the sighted to the non-sighted side.
6. Continue to encourage awareness of the nonsighted field until the patient can ultimately visualize the movement when the string is removed.

PERIPHERAL AWARENESS TRAINING WITH A MINUS LENS

Material: A minus lens between –3.00 and –10.00 D.

Goal: To make you aware of your environment.

Sequence of Activity:

1. Hold the minus lens at arm's length in front of your eye with the best sight and/or the largest field.
2. Move the lens closer to or farther from your eye until the clearest minified image is seen.
3. Identify objects in the environment based on their position.
4. Remove the lens and scan to verify the observation of object's position.
5. Walk safely through the environment, remembering where objects appeared to be.

Appendix A: Visual Acuity Conversions

Clinicians use various notations to describe distance and near visual acuities (VAs). Although these notations are generally not interchanged, clinicians occasionally convert one notation to another simply because they are more comfortable with a particular notation. Table A.1 shows the metric system for distance VAs and its corresponding values in the English system. Table A.2 shows how to convert a millimeter-sized target into M and point notation and M notation into point notation. In addition, conversion from M to Snellen notation is shown. This conversion can be used only if the clinician knows the distance for which the Snellen chart is calibrated (e.g., 16 in., 13 in.). It is most important, both at distance and near, to note the distance at which the test is performed and the size of the test target.

We have found one additional formula beneficial in attempting to evaluate uncommunicative patients:

$$\frac{\text{Height of object (ft)}}{\text{Distance object seen (ft)}} \times 13{,}760 = 20/$$

This form of acuity can be considered a visibility acuity, suggesting that a target can be seen but not necessarily identified. However, this acuity is a great starting point for any number of functional activities, especially for nonverbal patients [1].

Table A.1.

Metric	English
6/120	20/400
6/60	20/200
6/30	20/100
6/24	20/80
6/21	20/70
6/18	20/60
6/15	20/50
6/12	20/40
6/9	20/30
6/7.5	20/25
6/6	20/20

Table A.2.

mm × 0.7	=	M
mm × 5.5	=	point
M × 8	=	point
M × 50	=	20/Snellen (referred to the 40-cm test distance)

REFERENCE

1. Carter K. Comprehensive Preliminary Assessment of Low Vision. In R Jose (ed), Understanding Low Vision. New York: AFB Publishing, 1982;88.

Appendix B:
Basic Low Vision Optics

Jay M. Cohen

CLINICAL APPROACH TO LOW VISION OPTICS

Mastering the basic concepts of magnification and low vision optics will distinguish you from the doctor who merely provides the opportunity to try various optical devices. It allows more efficient delivery of care and guarantees that selection of the optical device is by intent rather than by chance.

For most practitioners, the term *low vision optics* conjures up murky images of complex and incomprehensible formulas. The aim of this appendix is to remove some of the mystique surrounding low vision optics and offer a simpler mathematical model that is more clinically relevant and can be immediately incorporated into your examination sequence. The use of optical formulas here is minimized and the discussion of mathematical concepts is restricted to those used in normal, everyday activities.

Although the mathematics and theory have been simplified, some parts (particularly the discussion on the way the different categories of optical devices work) are somewhat complicated. Read through those sections slowly and try to follow the examples. Once the basic concept is understood, your examination process will be streamlined and performed more quickly.

There are two distinct decision-making processes you face with every patient: (1) determining the appropriate power of the add, and (2) determining devices that can provide that power and be used for the tasks the patient wants to perform.

FINDING THE RIGHT ADD POWER

You must first understand what you are measuring and what you are attempting to accomplish in the testing sequence for low vision devices. Simply put, you are trying to reconcile two visual angles:

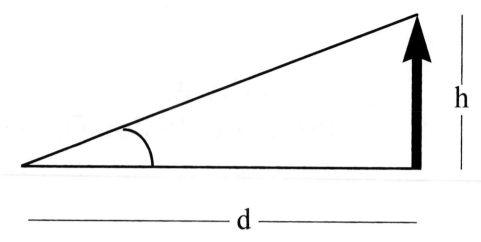

Figure B.1. Tangent of angle = h/d. This value is constant for the angle. (h = height of the object; d = distance from the eye.)

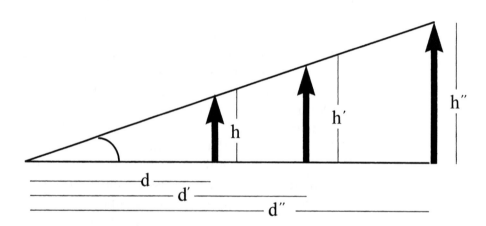

Figure B.2. h/d = h'/d' = h"/d". Any ratio representing this angle must equal h/d.

the patient's threshold angle of resolution (visual acuity) with the visual angle of the task demand (this is usually the desired print size the patient wants to be able to read). The goal is to make the object visible by magnifying the visual angle of the task demand so that it is at least as large or larger than the patient's threshold visual angle of resolution.

Because much of the discussion involves visual angles, it is appropriate to review some basic geometry. Visual angles are precise geometric units defined by the relationship between two factors: the height of the object (h) and the distance from the eye (d) (Figure B.1).

This relationship, h/d, is the tangent of the angle and is unique for each specific angle. Any combination of object height and object distance that generates a value equal to h/d will represent conditions of equal angular size (Figure B.2).

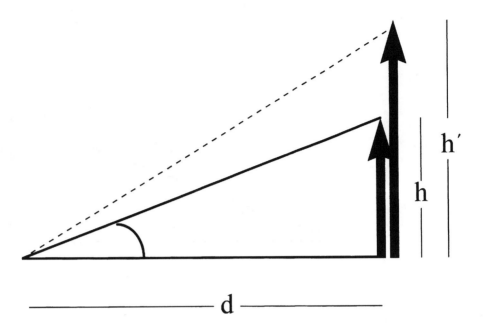

Figure B.3. h' > h, h'/d > h/d. Increasing the size of the object increases the size of the angle.

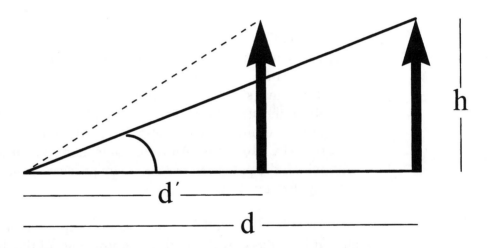

Figure B.4. d' < d, h/d' > h/d. Decreasing the distance increases the angle size.

When confronted with the clinical challenge of enlarging the visual angle of an object, three approaches can be taken:

1. Modify the object size while maintaining object distance. Since h is increased, h/d is increased. Clinical examples are the use of large print or a closed-circuit television (CCTV) at the patient's habitual working distance (Figure B.3).

2. Modify the object distance while maintaining object size. As d is decreased, h/d is increased. An example is moving closer to read a street sign (Figure B.4).

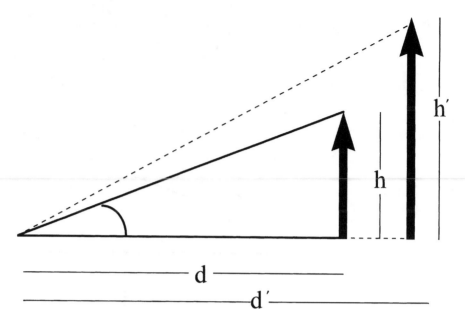

Figure B.5. h'/d' > h/d. When both object size and distance are altered, the angle size is increased only when the ratio h'/d' is greater than the original ratio h/d.

3. Finally, modify both object distance and object size. This is a little tricky because a positive gain in one parameter can be partially or wholly canceled out by a negative change in the other. Thus, doubling the object size while doubling the object distance results in no net gain in the size of the visual angle h'/d' = 2h/2d = h/d. The total change is determined by the ratio h'/d', which must be larger than the original value of h/d. An example is using a stand magnifier with which the patient views an enlarged image at an increased viewing distance (Figure B.5).

Applying this model clinically, the simple relationship between similar triangles of h/d = h'/d' and knowledge of the difference between what the patient can read and what the patient wants to read enables you to calculate the parameters that will allow patients to accomplish their goals.

The patient's basic reference angle h/d is determined by the visual acuity measurement. This is the smallest print the patient can read and represents a specific letter size (h) at a specific test distance (d). For objects to be seen, the ratio generated by the task demand, h'/d', must be greater than or equal to h/d. For example, suppose the patient is a college professor with two goals: to read 0.5 M manuscript print and to read computer-printed lecture notes at 50 cm (20 in.). You measure his reading acuity as 2 M at 40 cm (16 in.). For the first goal, the ratios h/d = h'/d' become 2 M/40 cm = 0.5 M/d', and d' = 0.5 × 40/2 = 10 cm. Holding the 0.5 M print at

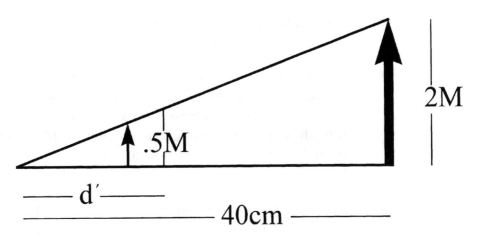

Figure B.6. Tangent of angle = h/d = h'/d' and 0.5/d' = 2/40, d' = 40 × 0.5/2 = 10 cm.

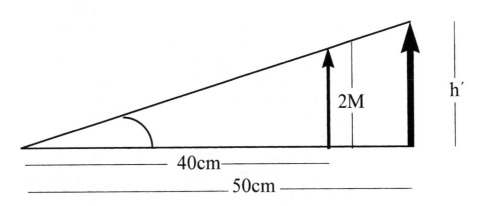

Figure B.7. Tangent of angle = h/d = h'/d', and h'/50 = 2/40, h' = 2 × 50/40 = 2.5 M.

10 cm subtends a visual angle equal to 2 M at 40 cm. For this working distance, a near add or accommodation of +10.00 D is required (Figure B.6).

For the second goal, the ratios become 2 M/40 cm = h'/50 cm, h' = 2 × 50/40, and h' = 2.5 M. He must print out his lecture notes in 2.5 M print to read them at the desired 50-cm (20 in.) distance. At 50 cm, the 2.5 M print will be as large as the 2 M print at 40 cm (Figure B.7).

The previous example demonstrates that you can manage the calculations using basic math concepts that are similar to those used when buying groceries. Few people are threatened by the following scenario: You go to the supermarket and oranges are four for $1. How many oranges can you get for $1.50? Most of us can mentally perform the calculation of x/$1.50 = 4/$1, and x = 4 × 1.5 = 6 oranges. Likewise, if oranges are four for $1, how much will one orange cost? The calculation is $x/1 = $1/4, and x = $1/4 = $0.25.

Clinically, the point of this lesson is to think of oranges rather than reciprocals of vision, and instead of buying fruit for dollars, you are buying magnification for diopters.

This leads to the next area of discussion, determining the dioptric power of the add. Diopters are the inverse of distance in meters. Once you have determined the working distance in meters that will provide adequate magnification of the task object, calculate its reciprocal. For example, 10 in. = 25 cm = 0.25 M, and 1/0.25 = 4.00 D; 13 in. = 33 cm = 0.33 M, and 1/0.33 M = 3.00 D; 1.6 in. = 4 cm = 0.04 M, and 1/0.04 = 25.00 D.

Once you are comfortable using this model, a modified method simply replaces distance with diopters in the original calculation of $h/d = h'/d'$. Diopter = $1/d$, so the formula now becomes $hD = h'D'$ and $D' = Dh/h'$. Put simply, this means the required add (D') for a particular object is equal to the add used for measuring the near acuity (D) times the ratio of the near acuity to the target print (h/h'). (The ratio h/h' is nothing more than the print magnification.)

Using the earlier example, acuity was 2 M at 40 cm and the patient wanted to be able to read 0.5 M print. A +2.50 D add or accommodation is needed for 40 cm and $D' = (2/0.5) \times 2.5 = 10.00$ D. For the 50-cm (20-in.) working distance, +2.00 D is required, and the necessary print size, therefore, is $2h' = 2.5 \times 2$ M, and $h' = 2.5$ M (see Figure B.7).

As long as you check that the working distance used for the acuity measurement corresponds to the add used, this second approach is probably simpler to use clinically, because it deals directly with diopters and requires only a single calculation.

Review the steps for determining the theoretic add necessary to achieve the appropriate magnification:

1. Determine specific patient goals by a thorough case history.
2. After a careful refraction, measure an accurate near acuity at the precise distance corresponding to the add or accommodation used.
3. Calculate the initial add for each goal by the relationship of $hD = h'D'$ (or $h/d = h'/d'$).

Some additional factors to keep in mind are as follows:

1. If reading is the patient's goal, then near acuity is best measured using continuous text cards rather than letter or isolated word cards.

2. M notation acuity is the preferred unit of measure for near acuity because of size consistency and simplification of calculations. "Normal" print is approximately 1 M. Since the goal of most patients is to read regular print, the math reduces to $hD = 1 \times D'$ or

D' = hD. The predicted add is equal to the add used for measuring the acuity times the acuity in M notation. For example, if the patient reads 4 M print with a +3.00 D add, reading 1 M print will require D' = 4 × 3 = 12.00 D.

    3. Use lighting similar to the patient's habitual lighting conditions.

    4. Modify the add through testing with actual printed materials such as newspapers, utility bills, books, and price tags. Keep a folder with selected materials in your office and ask the patient to bring samples of any special materials to be read.

FINDING THE BEST EQUIVALENT POWER OPTICAL AID

At this point, you have determined the power needed to magnify the task demand. The next step is to find the low vision device that provides that power in a way that is acceptable to the patient.

An acceptable device must meet the following criteria:

1. It must provide sufficient magnification.
2. It must meet the ergonomic demands of the task.
3. It must be reflective of the patient's self-image. In other words, the patient must be willing to use it.

The first criterion is the major topic of interest here. You must be able to differentiate devices that can generate sufficient magnification from those that cannot. You must then help the patient select the device that provides sufficient power and best meets the remaining criteria. Meeting the second criterion depends on understanding the patient history (see Chapter 2).

There are two factors to consider when deciding whether a device is strong enough for a patient's need—magnification and system dioptric power. The two factors are related but not synonymous.

Magnification is a relative measure based on the initial reference value and the desired final value. Clinically, it is the acuity divided by the goal (h/h'). System dioptric power, on the other hand, is an absolute value and is the same under all conditions. The term *system dioptric power*, denoted by the symbol F_s, refers to the value *Dh* (dioptric value of viewing distance × acuity) and represents the patient's threshold visual angle as discussed earlier.

An example should help clarify the distinction between the two terms. Patient A wants to read 1 M print and has a near acuity of 2 M using +5.00 D add at 20 cm (8 in.). Patient B also wants to read 1 M print and has an acuity of 3 M with a +2.50 D add at 40 cm (16 in.). Which patient needs more magnification and which patient needs the stronger lens?

Patient A reads 2 M print and wants to read 1 M print; therefore, 2 M/1 M or 2× magnification is necessary. F_s needed is +5.00 D × 2 = +10.00 D.

Patient B needs 3 M/1 M or 3× magnification and has an F_s of +2.5 × 3 = +7.50 D. Even though patient B needs one-and-a-half times the amount of magnification, he actually requires a weaker lens than patient A.

The reason for this apparent paradox is that magnification is comparing apples to oranges (i.e., different distances) while system dioptric power is comparing oranges to oranges (i.e., it compensates for different viewing distances). If patient B's acuity was measured at 20 cm—the same distance as that of patient A—he would see 1.5 M (D'h' = Dh, 5 × h = 2.5 × 3, and h = 1.5 M), demonstrating better acuity than patient A and thereby justifying the lower add. The magnification needed at this test distance becomes 1.5 M/1 M, or only 1.5×, but the F_s remains constant at 1.5 × +5.00 D = +7.50 D.

Adding to this confusion are the many unrelated types of magnification that you will be exposed to from other sources. The magnification you have been reading about is the total magnification of the baseline acuity the patient needs to see the desired task. There is also the manufacturer's magnification rating of magnifiers (usually based on one of two optical formulas: F/4 or F/4 + 1), which reflects the equivalent power of a magnifier's lens system, and transverse magnification (calculated by the optical formula u'/u = image distance/object distance) [1–3], which represents the optical enlargement of the image relative to the object.

Because of the variable value of magnification and the multiple uses of the term, use magnification only to help determine the dioptric need. Then use system dioptric power (F_s) to determine the equivalence of devices.

The visual angle generated by a system is based on the distance and size of the final object or image viewed. In determining the F_s, therefore, you must consider the location of the final image viewed (which is represented by the add or accommodative demand) and the magnification of the final object relative to the original object (which is the product of all the enlargement applications).

For example, for 1 M baseline print, what is the F_s of a patient with a +3.00 D add who sits 33 cm from a CCTV viewing 2 M print enlarged eight times on the screen? The first consideration is the location of the final image viewed—in this case it is the television screen at 33 cm or +3.00 D. The second consideration is the size of the final image. Relative to 1 M print, you have enlarged the image two ways—first by printing it two times larger and then by electronically enlarging it eight times. The total magnification is 2 × 8 = 16×. The F_s of this system is 3.00 D × 16 M = 48.00 D. This is the equivalent of trying to read 1 M print with a +48.00 D lens at approximately 2 cm.

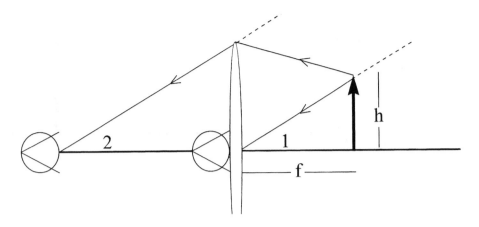

Figure B.8. Image at infinity. Tangent 1 = tangent 2 = h/f = hF. The angle size stays constant at all viewing distances.

To determine the F_s of a magnifier you must understand how the magnifier works. Although there are four major categories of optical devices—spectacles, hand-held magnifiers, stand magnifiers, and telescopes—there are only two optical conditions under which they operate: when the image is at infinity and when the image is closer than infinity.

IMAGE AT INFINITY

When the image is at infinity, the object of regard is at the focal point of the lens system. This means that light emerging from the lens is parallel and will subtend the same visual angle independent of the viewing distance from the lens (in other words, no matter how close or far you are from the lens, the image stays the same size). Therefore, if you can determine the visual angle of any one light ray, you will know the visual angle for every emerging light ray.

Fortunately, this is relatively easy to do. Any ray in object space that passes through the lens at its optical center will emerge in image space without deviation. If you take a ray from the top of the object and connect it to the lens at the optical axis, you have defined the angle in known quantities. The x-axis measurement (d) is, by definition, the focal length of the lens, f. The y-axis measurement (h) is, by definition, the object size. This means that when the image is at infinity, the visual angle exiting the system is equal to the familiar formula $h/d = h/f$ and $F_s = hF$, the dioptric power of the lens times the print size (Figure B.8).

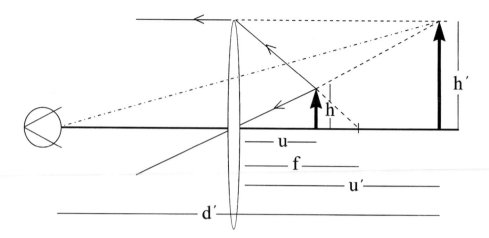

Figure B.9. Image not at infinity. Angle size = h'/d'. However, h'/u' = h/u, h' = hu'/u. u'/u = transverse magnification.

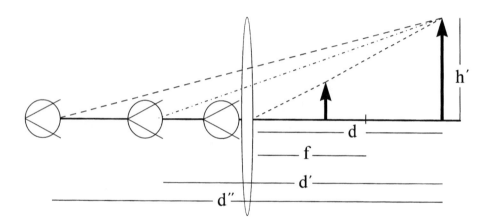

Figure B.10. Image not at infinity. Angle size varies with viewing distance. d < d' < d". Therefore, h'/d > h'/d' > h'/d".

IMAGE CLOSER THAN INFINITY

When the object of regard is closer than the focal point of the system, the virtual, enlarged image is at some finite distance behind it (Figure B.9). Even though the image is virtual, you must treat it like a real object in the sense that as you get closer and farther away from it the visual angle will increase and decrease, respectively (Figure B.10). Therefore, unlike the condition (i.e., image at infinity) in which the visual angle is constant, the visual angle is constantly changing as the patient moves relative to the magnifier. This complicates matters clinically, because you can have an optical system capable of providing variable amounts of power, and conditions of use play an important part in providing sufficient magnification.

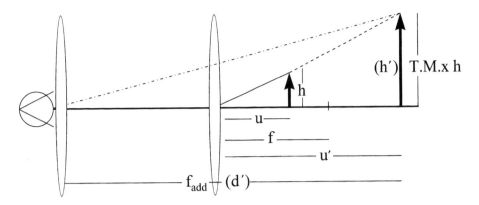

Figure B.11. Image not at infinity and angle size = h'/d'. However, h' = TM × h, and d' = f_{add}. Angle size = f_{add} × TM × h = F_{add} × TM × h. (TM = transverse magnification.)

The magnifier, once in place, provides a stable image relative to the lens. This image is a set distance from the lens and is of a specific size. The image distance is u' from the basic lens formula 1/f = 1/u' − 1/u, and the image size is the transverse magnification (u'/u) times the object size. However, the visual angle subtended by the image is not determined by the distance from the image to the lens, but rather by the distance from the image to the eye. This distance is the sum of the eye-to-lens distance and the lens-to-image distance. This distance also dictates the amount of accommodation or the power of the add needed to see the image clearly (Figure B.11).

The final visual angle of the system, therefore, is h'/d' = transverse magnification (TM) × object size/eye-to-image distance, and F_s = F_A × TM × h (power of add × magnified image size).

For example, if a stand magnifier enlarges an object 5×, then the patient viewing 1 M print using a +3.00 D add will have a F_s = +3.00 D × (5 × 1) = +15.00 D. If the patient now views the image with a +1.00 D add, F_s = +1.00 D × (5 × 1) = +5.00 D. Likewise, if the patient looks at 2 M print with the +3.00 D add, F_s = +3.00 D × (5 × 2) = +30.00 D.

The easiest way to find this information is to look it up in published charts that compile the optical characteristics of most commercially available magnifiers (see Appendix C). You can also ask your low vision device distributors if they provide such information. Another way is to measure these parameters yourself. This technique is beyond the scope of this chapter and is detailed elsewhere [1, 3].

A quick clinical technique that provides a ballpark value for stand magnifiers is to place the magnifier on the page and place plus lenses directly on the magnifier lens. Increase the power of the plus lenses until the first perceptible image blur occurs. (It is important that you view the image with your full-distance prescription

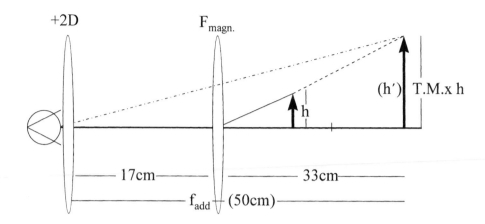

Figure B.12. Image not at infinity. Maximum add = u'. f_{add} = eye-to-image distance, which is the sum of the eye-to-lens distance and u'.

and that you are as close to the lenses as possible.) The most plus lens that provides a clear image gives you the approximate location of the image and allows you to estimate the transverse magnification as well as the ergonomic potential of the particular magnifier.

For example, if you find that a +3.00 D lens on top of the magnifier is the strongest lens used before the image starts blurring, the image is 33 cm (13 in.) behind the lens. Any spectacle the patient has with an add stronger than +3.00 D cannot be used with this magnifier and any weaker lens will have limitations on its working distance from the magnifier, defined by the focal length of the spectacle add minus the focal length of the maximum add. In this case, if the patient has a +2.00 D add, the patient must be 50 cm (20 in.) from the image. Because the image is 33 cm (13 in.) behind the magnifier lens, the patient must be 50 cm − 33 cm = 17 cm (7 in.) from the magnifier. Any target at a distance greater than 17 cm will be blurry (Figure B.12).

To estimate the transverse magnification, you must make use of the fact that when two lenses are in contact with each other, the total power is equal to the sum of the individual lens powers. In this case, assume the magnifier lens power is +20.00 D. However, we also know that F_s is equal to the F_A × TM. We know F_A = +3. Therefore, +3 × TM = +23.00 D and TM is approximately 23/3 or 7.67×. If the patient were to use a +2.00 D add, the F_s is +2 × 7.67 = +15.30 D.

A second approach to dealing with optical systems when the image is a finite distance away is to rely on the formula $F_{eq} = F_1 + F_2 − cF_1F_2$ (where F_{eq} = equivalent lens power, F_1 = magnifier, F_2 = spectacle add, and c = separation of F_1 and F_2 in meters). In the above example using +2.00 D add, F_{eq} = 20 + 2 − 0.17 × 2 × 20 = +15.20 D. Clinically, it is not practical to start measuring the separation between the lenses to calculate the F_{eq}; however, the formula can be used in a qualitative sense to provide information about F_{eq}.

Looking at the formula, you quickly note that only one variable—namely, c—is limited in the practical sense to between 0 and f_2, the focal length of the spectacle add. At c = 0, $F_{eq} = F_1 + F_2 + 0$, or the sum of the two lenses. This occurs when the magnifier is held up against the bifocal or reading lens. The power of F_{eq} will now get progressively weaker as c increases. At the other end of the range, c = f_2, (or in other words c = $1/F_2$), and $F_{eq} = F_1 + F_2 - (F_1 F_2/F_2) = F_2$. The separation between the lenses is the focal length of the add and the power is that of the add alone. The magnifier is touching the print and serves no useful purpose. A third key point in space is when c = f_1 (or c = $1/F_1$). At that position, $F_{eq} = F_1 + F_2 - [(F_1 + F_2)/F_1]$ or $F_{eq} = F_1$. When the separation is the focal length of the magnifier, the power is equal to that of the magnifier alone, and the spectacle add contributes nothing to the system. This point, f_1, is the critical dividing point in space.

If the magnifier is used with distance glasses, the material must be held at the focal point of the magnifier lens to create an image at infinity that can be seen clearly by the distance glasses. The power of the system is that of the magnifier, as discussed earlier in the section about the image at infinity. This relationship between the image and lens separation distance is the touchstone of whether it is worth using the magnifier with an add. As long as the separation of the lenses is between 0 and f_1, the F_{eq} will be greater than or equal to the power of the magnifier alone. As the separation increases in size from the focal length of the magnifier to the focal length of the add, the F_{eq} decreases from the power of the magnifier alone to that of the add alone.

The case of a patient who wears a bifocal with a +3.00 D add and uses a +10 magnifier illustrates this point. If the patient uses the magnifier with the distance part of the glasses, and the material at the focal point (10 cm) of the +10 magnifier, the patient has an F_{eq} of +10. Since the image is at infinity, the power is constant, regardless of the eye-to-lens separation. If the patient now chooses to use the bifocal segment and places the magnifier up against the spectacles (c = 0), then F_{eq} = 10 + 3 or 13.00 D. He gains +3.00 D in power over use of the magnifier alone with the distance prescription. If the patient now moves the magnifier 5 cm (2 in.) away, this is less than the focal length of the magnifier (10 cm), so he still ends up with a gain. The actual power is $10 + 3 - 0.5 \times 10 \times 3 = +11.50$.

If the patient moves the magnifier to 10 cm (4 in.), which is the focal length of the magnifier, the patient has reached the break-even point. The power is that of the magnifier alone ($F_{eq} = 10 + 3 - 0.5 \times 10 \times 3 = +10$). If he moves the magnifier to 20 cm, the separation is between the values f_1 and f_2, and therefore, F_{eq} will be between F_1

and F_2. (Actual $F_{eq} = 10 + 3 - 0.2 \times 10 \times 3 = +7.00$ D), so he sees better than with just the add, but not as well as using the magnifier with the distance portion of his glasses. Finally, if the patient holds the magnifier at 33 cm (13 in.)—the focal length of the add—F_{eq} is equal to only $+3$ ($F_{eq} = 10 + 3 - 0.3 \times 10 \times 3 = +3$), and it is a waste of time to use the magnifier.

The following list demonstrates how these theories apply to each of the four categories of optical devices.

1. *Spectacles.* Reading spectacles work with the print held at the focal point of the lens. The image is at infinity and F_s is the power of the lens. A +10 spectacle has a system power of +10.00 D, a + 20 spectacle is +20.00 D, and a 6× is +24.00 D. (With spectacles, × denotes F/4, so 6× = F/4 and F = 6 × 4 = +24.00 D.) Once you determine the F_s the patient needs, select a spectacle whose power is greater than or equal to F_s.

2. *Hand-held magnifiers.* Because they are hand held and can be placed anywhere in space, these magnifiers have two uses. In the simplest application they are used with distance spectacles and held above the print at the focal point of the lens. The image is at infinity, and similar to the spectacle, the magnifier lens provides F_s equal to the power of the lens itself. F_s remains constant regardless of the viewing distance. Select a trial hand-held magnifier with a power equal to or greater than the calculated F_s.

The second application is to use the hand-held magnifier with a near spectacle add. As long as the magnifier is less than its focal-length distance from the add, power will be greater than or equal to the power of the magnifier alone. Again, it is best to select a hand-held magnifier close in power to the calculated F_s and modify it based on patient response.

3. *Stand magnifiers.* These optical devices are the most difficult to control because the power of the magnifier lens has little to do with the F_s generated by the optical system. The two critical pieces of information needed for stand magnifiers are (1) where the image is located (maximum add), which tells you the range of add powers that can be used with this magnifier; and (2) the image magnification: F_s = spectacle add × image magnification × print size. Select a stand magnifier and spectacle add combination that provides the patient with an F_s equal to or greater than the calculated F_s.

4. *Telemicroscopes.* These devices are telescopes adapted for near. A telescope is a focal system that magnifies an incoming ray bundle from infinity without altering its vergence. When used at near, a plus reading lens is placed over the telescope objective lens to collimate the object for infinity. The power of the reading cap is related to the distance from the object to the telescope. Thus, an object 40 cm (16 in.) from the telescope needs a +2.50 D lens, while an object 33

cm (13 in.) away needs a +3.00 D lens. A second way to adapt a telescope for near is to increase the tube length of focusable design telescopes. Increasing the tube length increases the magnification; however, for most clinical situations this change is small enough to be ignored. The near-focused system can then be considered as the earlier case of a reading cap (the power of which is the inverse of the telescope-to-object distance) placed over the telescope objective.

The F_s of the telemicroscope is simply the power of the reading cap times telescopic magnification. So for a $4 \times$ TS with a +3.00 D cap, $F_s = 4 \times 3 = +12.00$ D. A 3× telescope with a +4.00 D cap will yield the same F_s of $3 \times 4 = +12.00$ D. The first example provides +12.00 D at a 33-cm (13-in.) working distance, and the second case provides the same at a 25-cm (10-in.) distance, as compared to a +12.00 D spectacle, which requires an 8.3-cm (3.3-in.) working distance. The advantage of the telemicroscope should now be obvious: It allows you to custom design an optical system for any distance needed. The disadvantage of these systems is that the field of view drops dramatically with increasing telescope power.

CASE STUDIES

Patient 1

Patient 1 is an 89-year-old woman with a history of macular degeneration. She wishes to read newspapers, magazines, and her mail, all of which are approximately 1 M print. The patient has best-corrected distance visual acuity of 20/200 and, when tested at 33 cm with a +3.00 D add, can read 4 M continuous text print with reasonable fluency.

The first step is to establish the system power needed to meet the patient's goal of reading 1 M print. She reads 4 M print with a +3.00 D add; therefore, +3.00 D × 4 M = D' × 1 M, and D' = +12.00 D. Start with +12.00 D trial spectacle add. The +12.00 D add allows the patient to read 1 M print at 8.3 cm (3.3 in.) with some difficulty and newspaper with great difficulty. You now increase the strength of the add to fine tune the best lens. You discover that a +14.00 D add enables the patient to read a newspaper with moderate proficiency and standard typewritten print with great proficiency. Further increasing the add does not improve performance. With a good reading lamp, the same performance is achieved with the +12.00 D add. The patient strongly objects to the close working distance of the spectacle and refuses to accept the device.

You must show the patient other options that, based on the spectacle trial, should be in the +12.00 D to +14.00 D power range. You find that a +12.00 D illuminated hand-held magnifier works well. It permits even newspaper to be read with ease; however, the patient complains of difficulty maintaining focus after a few minutes of reading.

You now want to demonstrate stand magnifiers, which provide a stable base for prolonged reading tasks. You must select magnifiers that are capable of generating at least a +12.00 D system power, preferably with the +3.00 D add the patient already has. (Otherwise a new near add for use with the magnifier must be prescribed.) Ideally, you are looking for a stand magnifier with a transverse magnification greater than 4× and a maximum add of at least +3.00 D. Two readily available stand magnifiers meet this description (see Appendix C): (1) the Selsi Jupiter Loupe with a transverse magnification of 3.9× and a maximum add of 4.25 D, and (2) the COIL Raylite 3.9× with a TM of 4.1× and maximum add of 3.50 D. Patient reaction to these magnifiers should guide you in modifying the selection. In this case, however, the patient is pleased with both magnifiers. She prefers the COIL 3.9× because it has a built-in light and is better for reading newspaper.

She is slightly dissatisfied with the working distance of 4 cm from the lens (33 cm focal length for +3.00 D add – 29-cm lens-to-image distance = 4 cm) and requests any device that may permit her to read at her habitual distance. This requires a telemicroscope with a +3.00 D cap to obtain the 33-cm (13-in.) distance. Since she needs F_s = +12.00 D to 14.00 D and F_s = magnification × reading cap, this requires a telescope power of +12/+3 = 4× to +14/+3 = 4.67×. You try a 4× telescope. The patient has a great deal of difficulty localizing the print and is unhappy with the field restriction of the telescope. She declines further trial with telescopes.

At this point you are ready to wrap things up. You recommend the +12.00 D illuminated hand magnifier for portability and short-term reading tasks, such as reading price tags, mail, and scanning. You also recommend the 3.9× illuminated stand for longer reading tasks. You must stress that she should use her reading add with the stand magnifier and may find that a reading stand to hold the material will improve comfort.

This idealized case illustrates several points discussed earlier and demonstrates a systematic approach to the selection of low vision devices rather than the shotgun approach used by those unfamiliar with optics. It streamlines the testing process by targeting low vision devices with a high probability of success. To be successful, this approach requires a knowledge of how the devices work and the properties of the magnifiers in your stock. As you provide more low vision care, your familiarity with devices will increase but, until that time, it is convenient to mark the trial magnifiers with their lens power and the transverse magnification and maximum add for the stand magnifiers.

Patient 2

Patient 2 is a 27-year-old male with a history of congenital cataracts. He is aphakic and wears a contact lens correction. He is enrolled in a graduate chemistry program and is seeking help for two problems. He must read the markings on pipettes held under the laboratory hood and the fine-print precautions on the chemical jar labels. The pipettes have markings of approximately 1.5 M and are held 67 cm (27 in.) away. The jar labels have print size of approximately 0.5 M.

The patient is currently corrected with contact lenses to 20/160 in each eye and uses a pair of +12.00 D half eyes for fluent reading of 1 M print. Refraction yields no change in the contact lens correction, and with a +2.50 D add at 40 cm, the patient reads 3.2 M print and 4 M continuous text.

To determine the power necessary for each task, use the formula hD = h'D'. For the pipette marking, a number identification task, this is equal to 2.5×3.2 M = D' $\times$ 1.5 M, D = $2.50 \times 3.2/1.5$ = +5.30 D. Round up to +5.50 D. For the 0.5 M continuous label text, a reading task, this is +2.5 $\times$ 4.0 M = D' $\times$ 0.5 M = $2.5 \times 4/0.5$ = +20.00 D.

The ergonomic demands of reading the pipettes at 67 cm require a system that will leave the hands free and provide F_s = +5.50 D at 67 cm (+1.50 D distance). The only device that meets both criteria is a head-borne telescope. Since F_s = magnification $\times$ reading cap, the telescopic power needed is +5.5 = M $\times$ +1.5, and M = 5.5/1.5 = 3.67$\times$. In terms of commercially available systems, this must be rounded up to 4$\times$ or down to 3$\times$. The 4$\times$ telescope with a +1.50 D cap will provide F_s = +6.00 D, slightly more than predicted, while the 3$\times$ telescope will require a +2.00 D cap to provide the same power (+5.5 = 3 $\times$ D, and D = +1.83 D, rounded up to +2.00 D). The patient feels the shortened working distance would not be adequate for the task. A trial with the 4$\times$ telescope allows the patient to perform the task satisfactorily.

Questioning the patient reveals the second task of reading labels is short term and required only intermittently. You decide, therefore, that this need will best be served with a small magnifier used while looking over the half eyes. Based on the predicted power for continuous text, you try a +20.00 D magnifier, which works well. Your recommendations to the patient, therefore, are a spectacle-mounted 4$\times$ telescope system, with a +1.50 D cap and a +20.00 D hand magnifier.

Summary

These two cases are modified from actual patient encounters to help illustrate the clinical decision-making process in action.

1. Determine the patient's need
2. Calculate the power needed to meet each objective
3. Refine the power through actual testing
4. Select appropriately powered devices

5. Guide the patient in the selection of the device that best meets the patient's needs

Finding the device that best meets your patient's needs involves the consideration of many factors. These include obvious physical specifications as well as more subtle psychological ones. For example, although a +6.00 D spectacle or hand-held magnifier allows Patient 2 to read the pipette markings, they are inappropriate, because the spectacles require too short a working distance and the hand magnifier does not leave the hands free. A gooseneck magnifier of the same power, however, might be a consideration. Patient 1 demonstrates some of the psychological factors of low vision testing. For long-term reading tasks, spectacles generally provide the widest field of view and are usually the most practical option. However, many patients cannot accept the close working distance, often because of self-image, and will opt instead for hand-held devices that may not offer a significantly longer working distance.

The key characteristics of each type of optical system are as follows (see Chapter 4 for a review):

1. *Spectacles* leave the hands free and provide the widest field of view for each particular power. They permit binocular correction and can be prescribed as full field, half-eyes, or bifocals. It is usually the best device for long-term reading tasks if the patient can tolerate the close working distance and the distance blur when looking beyond the focal range of the lens.

2. *Hand-held magnifiers* provide great flexibility in working distance and are relatively inexpensive. They do, however, tie up one hand and require extensive scanning, making them fatiguing for long-term tasks. The hand-held magnifier is typically used as a portable, short-term spotting device.

3. *Stand magnifiers* provide a stable optical image and facilitate scanning by maintaining the lens position. They are somewhat bulky and require the use of an appropriate add.

Illuminated stands are readily available and are a boon to patients requiring elevated light levels. The problem with stand magnifiers is knowing what exact system power is being generated in each instance. Stands are good general purpose magnifiers.

4. *Telescopes* allow system power to be generated at any desired working distance. They are expensive, and because of field and spatial constraints they are often difficult for patients to adapt to. Telescopes are used when task parameters require an extended working distance. When adapted for near tasks, task demands usually require the telescope to be spectacle mounted.

Selection of the best option is based on task demands, patient performance, and patient comfort. You have been given a framework for delivering low vision care. The critical step is to transfer this theory into clinical practice by using this book as your guide. The only way to do it is to jump in and start working with patients. The mathematics have been presented as simply as possible, but keeping a pocket calculator or cheat sheet on your desk should help until the process becomes automatic and you can do the calculations in your head.

PROBLEMS

Here are some sample problems (and their solutions) to get your thinking in gear and test how well you have picked up the concepts.

1. A patient reads 6.4 M continuous text at 33 cm (13 in.) using a +3.00 D add. What is the system power you will need if the patient wants to read 1 M continuous text?
2. What if the patient in problem 1 wants to read 0.6 M?
3. A patient who is 2.00 D myopic can read 2.5 M print at 20 cm while wearing +3.00 D reading spectacles. What system power will the patient need to read 1 M text?
4. A patient needs to read the 0.5 M print footnotes found on the bottom of her textbook page. You decide to try a stand magnifier. What parameters should you look for in a magnifier if the patient reads the 1.25 M text with a +4.00 D add?
5. The patient is a building superintendent whose responsibilities include checking the boiler's pressure gauge once a week. The closest distance that he can easily reach to see the gauge is about 1 meter. The patient's best-corrected acuity is 20/70, and he can read 1.5 M print at 40 cm (16 in.) with a +2.50 D add. If the numbers on the gauge are about 2 M print, what optical system might you try to solve the problem?
6. An emmetropic patient uses a +2.00 D add with a stand magnifier to read his 2 M large-print books. The transverse magnification of the magnifier is 4×. He wishes to know if he will be able to read 1 M print price tags with a +20.00 D hand magnifier he recently purchased. What do you tell him?
7. A patient uses a +20.00 D hand magnifier and wants to know if she will see better using it with her +4.00 D reading glasses instead of her distance glasses. What advice can you give her?
8. Another patient presently reads using a +5.00 D add. A friend just gave her a +10.00 D hand magnifier, and she

wants to know if it will help her see the print better. What do you tell her?

9. A patient can read 3.2 M with a +2.50 D add and would like to read 0.8 M. Which of the following options are appropriate: (a) +10 hand magnifier, (b) +12.00 D spectacle add, (c) a stand magnifier with a +2.00 D maximum add and 5.5× transverse magnification, (d) a 4× telescope with a +2.50 D cap, or (e) a +2.50 D add with a CCTV to 6× magnification?

ANSWERS

The solutions are based on the formula hD = h'D'.

1. The patient reads 6.4 M print with a +3.00 add. The threshold visual angle is $6.4 \times 3 = 19.2$ to read 1 M print. hD = h'D' or $19.2 = 1 \times D'$ and D' = +19.20 D (round up to +20.00 D).

2. If the goal is to be able to read 0.6 M print, hD = h'D' becomes $19.2 = 0.6 \times D'$ and D' = +32.00 D.

3. The patient is 2.00 D myopic and is wearing a +3.00 D spectacle for a total add of +5.00 D. Because he reads 2.5 M print, hD = $2.5 \times 5 = 12.5$. To read 1 M print, hD = h'D', $12.5 = 1 \times D'$, and D' = +12.50 D.

4. The patient can read 1.25 M print with a +4.00 D add. hD = $1.25 \times 4 = 5$. Because she wishes to read 0.5 M print, the system power needed is hD = h'D', $5 = 0.5 \times D'$ and D' = 10.00 D. The stand magnifier must provide +10.00 D using the patient's +4.00 D add. Because the power of a stand magnifier is transverse magnification times the add, in this case $+10 = TM \times +4$ and TM = 10/4 = 2.5×. You need a stand magnifier with transverse magnification of at least 2.5× and a maximum add of at least +4.00 D.

5. Your patient has a threshold visual angle represented by hD = $1.5 \times 2.5 = 3.75$. The task demand represents a visual angle of h'D' = $2 \times 1 = 2$. Because of the required working distance, a telescope will provide the best option for this task. Because it is a short-term and very intermittent spotting task, a hand-held telescope is probably the most suitable choice. The magnification required is M × 2 = 3.75 M = 3.75/2 = 1.87× (round up to 2×). Your initial test device should be a 2× telescope with a +1.00 D cap or add. A second option, if the patient is tall enough, is to use a hand-held magnifier: hD = h'D', $3.75 = 2 \times D'$, D' = +1.875 D (round up to +2.00 D). A +2.00 D lens held 50 cm away (f = 50 cm, total distance = 1 M) should provide sufficient power to accomplish the goal.

6. The patient reads 2 M print with 4× TM and a +2.00 add. hD = (4 × 2) × 2 = 16. He wishes to read 1 M print with a +20.00 D hand magnifier h'D' = 1 × 20 = 20. Because h'D' > hD (20 > 16), he should be able to read 1 M print with the magnifier.

7. As long as the separation of the +4.00 D add and the magnifier is less than 5 cm (2 in.), the magnifier focal length, the system power will be greater than +20.00 D (the system power when the magnifier is used with only the distance correction). Therefore, you can tell her she will see better as long as the hand magnifier is no more than 2 in. from the reading glasses. Otherwise she should use her distance glasses.

8. The answer is yes. The worst she can do is hold the magnifier 20 cm (8 in.) from the near add, which results in a system power equal to the add itself (+5.00 D). Any other lens separation or use of the magnifier with the distance glasses will result in a system power greater than +5.00 D. Thus using the magnifier with the add will always result in a stronger power than use of the add alone.

9. hd = 3.2 × 2.5 = 8. For 0.8 M, h'D' = hD or 0.8D' = 8, D' = 8/0.8 = +10.00 D. Any system providing +10.00 D or greater power should be satisfactory. Therefore, all five options should provide sufficient magnification. F_s for (a) 10, (b) 12, (c) 2 × 5.5 = 11 (note that the patient cannot use his +2.50 D add with option C because the maximum add is only +2.00 D), (d) 4 × 2.5 = 10, and (e) 6 × 2.5 = 15.

REFERENCES

1. Bailey IL, Bullimore MA, Greer RB, Mattingly WB. Low vision magnifiers—their optical parameters and methods for prescribing. Optom Vis Sci 1994:71;689.

2. Cole RG. A Functional Approach to the Optics of Low Vision Devices. In RG Cole, BP Rosenthal (eds), Remediation and Management of Low Vision. St. Louis: Mosby, 1996;139.

3. Nowakowski RW. Primary Low Vision Care. East Norwalk, CT: Appleton & Lange, 1994.

Appendix C:
The Equivalent Viewing Distance System of Magnification Rating: A Rational Approach to Prescribing Magnifiers

Ian L. Bailey

EDITOR'S NOTE

In conjunction with Mattingly International, Dr. Ian Bailey has developed a system that codes the magnification of optical devices. This system allows the clinician to maintain the comparable magnification when using different types of low vision devices. It provides a more scientific and effective approach to prescribing such devices. The equivalent viewing distance (EVD) is the optical parameter that allows this direct comparison. This appendix includes a short description of the EVD system, along with some basic definitions, and, most importantly, a series of charts that allows the clinician to look up the EVD of magnifiers being considered for a given patient. The clinician can use the charts provided here to make an individualized chart for the office or clinic, including only those devices most often prescribed.

THE EQUIVALENT VIEWING DISTANCE SYSTEM

Some questions you must ask yourself when considering a specific low vision device follow:

- What image am I asking the patient to look at?
- Where and how big is this image?

- How far away is the image?
- Will the image be in focus?
- How big is it compared to the original?
- What is the enlargement ratio?
- What will the patient be able to see?
- What are the smallest details the patient can see?

These questions are most easily answered when magnifying effects are expressed as EVD.

> EVD = Distance at which the original object would subtend an angle that is equal to the angle subtended by the image at the observer's eye.
>
> EVD = actual viewing distance ÷ enlargement ratio

Examples:

- A closed-circuit television video magnifier enlarges image 10×
- Viewing this screen from 100 cm, the EVD = 10 cm
- Viewing this screen from 25 cm, the EVD = 2.5 cm
- If screen magnification is 5×, viewing from 25 cm, EVD = 5 cm

These examples illustrate that the same system can provide very different levels of magnification and, more importantly, different systems with the same EVD provide the same resolution.

> **Determining the EVD Required to Meet a Patient's Needs**
>
> 1. Set a resolution goal. For example, to read 0.8 M print (6.3 point, or telephone-book print).
> 2. Determine resolution limit when the acuity chart is at a known distance. The chart should be in satisfactory focus (not necessarily ideal focus). Resolution limit (smallest print read) and viewing distance should be noted.
>   Example: Patient with +2.50 D add reads 4 M print (32 point) at 25 cm. Focus seems fine. (+1.50 D add is not needed because low vision patients are usually less sensitive to blur.)
> 3. Calculate the EVD required to accomplish the desired task.
>   Example: A patient who reads 4.0 M print at 25 cm and wants to read 0.8 M print needs to move five times closer (4/0.8 = 5) (i.e., from 25 to 5 cm). Required EVD is 5 cm.
> 4. From the tables or your calculations, choose the most convenient system that gives required EVD or closer.

The following systems provide an EVD of 5 cm:

- A +20.00 D spectacle lens addition: Focuses at 5 cm.
- A +20.00 D hand-held magnifier, used to give image at infinity: Material held 5 cm from lens and parallel rays enter eye as though emanating from 5 cm away.
- Video magnifier at 40 cm with 8× enlargement: An image enlarged 8× at 40 cm is the same as moving the initial object 8× closer than 40 cm, or 40/8 = 5 cm.
- Stand magnifier giving eye-to-image distance of 30 cm and enlargement of 6×: The image magnified 6× at 30 cm is the same as moving the initial object 6× closer than 30 cm, or 30/6 = 5 cm.
- A 4× afocal telescope with a +5.00 D cap to focus for 20 cm: This is an image at 20 cm magnified 4× by the telescope. This is the same as moving the initial object 4× closer than 20 cm, or 20/4 = 5 cm.

With any of the above systems, it is as though the patient had the original object at 5 cm from the eye while having the required accommodation or addition to gain clear focus (Figure C.1).

The tables at the end of this appendix list optical parameters of low vision magnifiers based on measurements made by Ian Bailey, Mark Bullimore, Robert Greer, and Kuang-mon Tuan of the Low Vision Clinic at University of California, Berkeley. This project received support from Mattingly International.

An example of how to use these tables follows. Working through this example will show you how valuable these tables can be in helping you to more effectively prescribe low vision devices.

EXAMPLE

The patient requires an EVD of 6 cm or less to read print of the required size. Assume that the patient will choose to place the eye at a moderate distance ($z = 10$ cm) from the lens. Go to major column ($z = 10$ cm), consider EVD, eye-to-image distance, and field size. Look at magnifiers giving EVD of 6.0 cm or a bit less (5- to 6-cm range). The table lists eight illuminated magnifiers in this range (from Pike 5N to COIL 6289). Their eye-to-image distances range from 21 to 60 cm. One (21 cm) is unsatisfactory for an add of +2.50 D. If an add of +4.00 D is required, two image distances (59.1 and 60.4 cm) would probably be too remote. The field of view can be approximated by the formula:

Field width = Lens width × (EVD/eye-to-lens distance)

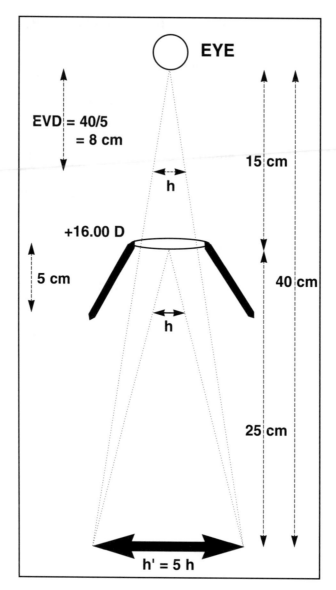

Figure C.1. Optics diagram. A thin +16.00 D lens gives an image distance of 25 cm (−4.00 D) when the object distance is 5 cm (−20.00 D). The enlargement ratio is 5×. Here, the eye is placed 15 cm above the lens. The 5× enlarged image is viewed from 40 cm (i.e., 15 + 25). Thus, equivalent viewing distance (EVD) = 40/5 = 8 cm. The angle subtended by the image is equal to the angle the object would subtend at a viewing distance of 8 cm. (h = object height; h' = image height.)

Because patients generally prefer larger fields, two of the systems have a field of view of 35 mm and 26 mm.

Note

From the eight magnifiers under consideration, imagine we chose the Pike 5 NB/NE 5× Illuminated (EVD = 6 cm if z = 10 cm). If the patient moves close to the Pike 5× (z = 2.5 cm), EVD becomes 4.9 cm and the field is larger. If patient moves back (25 cm), EVD and eye-to-image distance both increase and the field decreases. Using the tables in this manner allows you to provide the correct device and the optimum conditions to use it.

When prescribing hand-held magnifiers, two options exist.

1. **The magnifier is held remote from the eye.** If the eye-to-lens distance is longer than the focal length of magnifier, the patient should use distance glasses (or relax accommodation). Then EVD equals focal length of magnifier. The field will be smaller than the width of the magnifier lens.

Field width = Lens width × [(focal length)/(eye-to-lens distance)]

2. **The magnifier is held close to the eye.** The patient will gain some advantage by using a bifocal add but only if the eye-to-lens distance is shorter than the focal length of magnifier. When the magnifier and reading add are touching one another, the power of the system is the power of the magnifier plus the power of the add. The EVD will equal the focal length of the magnifier (or shorter). When the lens is held close to the eye, the field becomes larger than the width of the magnifier lens.

PRISM READERS

Basic Principles

Prism readers and binocular loupes usually impose close working distances. Close working distances create high convergence demands and the difference between the near interpupillary distance (NPD) and distance PD (DPD) can become substantial. Ready-made prism-reader spectacles and binocular loupes incorporate prism or decenter the lenses to minimize or control the convergence demand.

To simply place the optical centers at the near PD, the separation between optical centers should be

$$NPD = DPD\ [W/(W + z)]$$

where W is the working distance (in millimeters) from the spectacle plane and z is the distance from the spectacle plane to the center of eye rotation (= 27 mm).

With this amount of decentration, the convergence required will be the same as it would be without spectacles. That is, the lenses neither increase nor decrease the convergence demand.

An approximation for a quick estimation of the required decentration is

$$Decentration = 1.5\ (add\ power)$$

(i.e., DPD − NPD = 1.5 [working distance in diopters]).

Ready-Made Prism Readers

Most ready-made prism readers are labeled with their lens power (in diopters) and a prism value (prism diopters) that indicates how much base-in prism is incorporated into each lens.

Typically, the amount of prism is two greater than the lens power (e.g., +10.00 D, 12Δ; +6.00 D, 8Δ). One can think of the prism as being used partly to provide the decentration effect appropriate for the close working distance and partly to give a small amount of additional decentration to reduce the convergence demand.

Unfortunately, the optical parameters of prism readers are not usually fully specified. There is no information given about the assumed PD of the user and consequently the specifications of prism become vague and uncertain. Another problem with prism readers is that they have thick, tilted lenses. The patient's line of sight will pass through the thick lens at an oblique angle and often at a point that is significantly displaced with respect to the optical center. The exact calculation of prism effects and lens power effects requires dealing with oblique off-axis rays through thick lenses.

Convergence Demand for an Emmetrope

For prism readers, placing the object in the midline plane so that it is in the focal plane of both lenses will give rise to images at infinity for both the right and left eyes. These images at infinity are significantly separated and this means that the eyes must converge to fuse. The angle of required convergence is determined by the angle of the rays that join the object point to the anterior nodal points of the lenses. All rays originating from the object leave the lens as an emerging beam of parallel rays. A patient with a wider PD effectively uses rays that are more external within the emerging beams from the right and left lenses. The narrow PD patient uses rays that are more internal within the emerging beams.

The angle of convergence is the same regardless of PD. The point to which the eyes must converge does depend on the patient's PD. A narrower PD means a closer point of convergence; a wider PD means a more remote point of convergence.

SUGGESTED READING

Bailey IL. Locating the image in stand magnifiers. Optom Monthly 1981;72(6):22.

Bailey IL. Locating the image in stand magnifiers—an alternative method. Optom Monthly 1983;74:48t.

Bullimore MA, Bailey IL . Stand magnifiers—an evaluation of new optical aids from COIL. Optom Vis Sci 1989;66:766.

Bailey IL. Magnification of the problem of magnification. Optician 1984;187:14.

Bailey IL. Equivalent viewing power or magnification. Which is Fundamental? Optician 1984;188:33

Bailey IL. The Optometric Examination of the Elderly Patient. In AA Rosenbloom, MW Morgan (eds), Vision and Aging (2nd ed). Boston: Butterworth–Heinemann, 1992;200.

Bailey IL. Verifying near vision magnifiers. Part I. Optom Monthly 1981;72(1):42.

Bailey IL. Verifying near vision magnifiers. Part II. Optom Monthly 1981;72(2):34.

Bailey IL, Loshin D. Hand held magnifiers. Rehabil Optom 1984;1:29.

Freed B. A new method for the measurement of transverse magnification. Initial results in 21 selected stand magnifiers. J Vis Rehabil 1987;1(2):47.

TABLE 1 Illuminated Stand Magnifiers – Optical parameters

Manufacturer ID #	Descriptions	Illum code	Adjust	Lens size mm	Fe D.	l' cm	ER x	z=2.5 EVD	ey/im	fld	z=10.0 EVD	ey/im	fld	z=25 EVD	ey/im	fld	EVD-EVP
Mattingly 22x Ill a	22x Illum	be ih		17	66.4	####	####	1.5	####	10	1.5	####	3	1.5	####	1	
Peak 1996L	30x Illum	b i		8	120.4	10.0	13.0	1.0	12.5	3	1.5	20.0	1	2.7	35.0	1	1.6cm-63D
Mattingly 22x Ill b	22x Illum	be ih		17	66.4	21.3	15.1	1.6	23.8	11	2.1	31.3	4	3.1	46.3	2	
Eschenbach 1557	12.5x -46D Illum	be 1h		30	47.6	42.4	21.6	2.1	44.9	25	2.4	52.4	7	3.1	67.4	4	
Eschenbach 1557	12.5x/40, Illum	be hi		30	46.9	49.7	24.3	2.1	52.2	26	2.5	59.7	7	3.1	74.7	4	2.5cm-40D
Eschenbach 1550-1/204/3	10x-36D illum	he ih		35	36.4	63.3	24.0	2.7	65.8	38	3.1	73.3	11	3.7	88.3	5	
Peak 2023	15x Illum	be ih		18	45.8	16.1	8.4	2.2	18.6	16	3.1	26.1	6	4.9	41.1	4	
Eschenbach 1550	10x/40, 38D, Illum, scale	be hi		35	37.5	34.2	13.8	2.7	36.7	37	3.2	44.2	11	4.3	59.2	6	3.2cm-32D
COIL 5212/5212-10	12x-44D Hi-power Illum	bre ih		34	35.4	18.2	7.4	2.8	20.7	38	3.8	28.2	11	5.8	43.2	8	
COIL 5210/5210-10	10x-36D Hi-power illum	bre ih		36	30.7	25.0	8.7	3.2	27.5	46	4.0	35.0	15	5.8	50.0	8	4.0cm-25D
Peak 1966	10 Illum	be ih		26	29.2	22.4	7.5	3.3	24.9	34	4.3	32.4	11	6.3	47.4	7	
Eschenbach 1551	7x/55, 28D Illum	be hi		35	27.2	31.5	9.6	3.5	34.0	50	4.3	41.5	15	5.9	56.5	8	
Eschenbach 1551-1/204/3	7x-24D illum	be ih		35	24.1	65.0	16.7	4.1	67.5	57	4.5	75.0	16	5.4	90.0	8	
COIL 5228/5228-10	8x-28D Hi-power	bre ih		44	23.7	67.5	17.0	4.1	70.0	73	4.6	77.5	20	5.4	92.5	10	
Schweizer 162	8x flashlight mag	b ih		27	25.9	28.3	8.3	3.7	30.8	40	4.6	38.3	13	6.4	53.3	7	
Pike 7NB/7NE	7x Illum	be i		33	26.5	22.0	6.8	3.6	24.5	47	4.7	32.0	15	6.9	47.0	9	
COIL 5226/5226-10	6x-20D Hi-power	bre ih		50	23.7	41.5	10.8	4.1	44.0	81	4.8	51.5	24	6.1	66.5	12	
Eschenbach 1552-1/204/3	6x-20D illum	be ih		50	22.2	51.9	12.5	4.3	54.4	87	4.9	61.9	25	6.1	76.9	12	
COIL 6289	Raylite 24 24.2/7.1x	be ih		35	24.1	24.4	6.9	3.9	26.9	55	5.0	34.4	18	7.2	49.4	10	5.0cm-20D
COIL 5289	8x-28D Raylite 70	be ih		36	23.4	25.1	6.9	4.0	27.6	58	5.1	35.1	18	7.3	50.1	11	
Eschenbach 1552	6x/100, 23D, Illum	be hi		47	22.6	31.0	8.0	4.2	33.5	79	5.1	41.0	24	7.0	56.0	13	
Schweizer 1840	8x Leuchtlupe	b i		36	20.5	29.7	7.1	4.5	32.2	65	5.6	39.7	20	7.7	54.7	11	
Schweizer 190	8x, 28D, modular	be h		35	23.9	11.4	3.7	3.7	13.9	52	5.8	21.4	20	9.8	36.4	14	
Schweizer 190	8X-28D illum modular	be h	tilt	35	23.9	11.1	3.6	3.7	13.6	52	5.8	21.1	20	9.9	36.1	14	
Eschenbach 1553-3	5x-16D illum	be ih		60	18.4	50.4	10.3	5.1	52.9	124	5.9	60.4	35	7.3	75.4	18	
Pike 5NB/NE	5x Illum	be i		43	18.8	30.1	6.7	4.9	32.6	84	6.0	40.1	26	8.3	55.1	14	
COIL 6279	Raylite 18 17.7D/5.4x	be ih		44	18.2	33.3	7.1	5.1	35.8	89	6.1	43.3	27	8.2	58.3	15	6.3cm-16D
Schweizer 191	6x, 20D, modular	be h		55	18.6	12.2	3.3	4.5	14.7	99	6.8	22.2	37	11.4	37.2	25	
COIL 5279	6x-20D Raylite 50	be ih		47	17.9	13.3	3.4	4.7	15.8	88	6.9	23.3	32	11.3	38.3	21	
Schweizer 191	6X-20D illum modular	be h	tilt	55	18.1	12.5	3.2	4.6	15.0	102	6.9	22.5	38	11.6	37.5	25	
Eschenbach 1554-1/204/3	4x-12D illum	be ih		70	14.8	83.3	13.4	6.4	85.8	180	7.0	93.3	49	8.1	108.3	23	
Schweizer 149	6x-20D illum mag	b i		53	15.9	20.7	4.3	5.4	23.2	114	7.1	30.7	38	10.6	45.7	22	
Eschenbach 1525-1/204/3	8x Illum	be ih		50	16.7	13.3	3.2	4.9	15.8	98	7.2	23.3	36	11.9	38.3	24	
COIL 6269	Raylite 15 14.6D/4.7x	be ih		44	14.9	25.2	4.7	5.8	27.7	103	7.4	35.2	33	10.6	50.2	19	
Eschenbach 1554	4x/180, 16D, Illum	be hi		65	14.9	18.9	3.8	5.6	21.4	146	7.6	28.9	49	11.5	43.9	30	
COIL 5259	4x-15.6D Raylite 34	be ih		47	14.1	23.2	4.3	6.0	25.7	113	7.8	33.2	37	11.3	48.2	21	
Schweizer 150/150H	5x illum	be ih		55	14.3	13.1	2.9	5.4	15.6	119	8.0	23.1	44	13.2	38.1	29	8cm-12.5D
Eschenbach 1526-1/204/3	4x illum	be ih		60	13.6	17.8	3.4	5.9	20.3	142	8.1	27.8	49	12.5	42.8	30	
Schweizer 192	5x, 16D, modular	be h		60	14.1	12.2	2.7	5.4	14.7	130	8.1	22.2	49	13.7	37.2	33	
Schweizer 161	5x flashlight mag	b ih		58	13.5	17.5	3.4	6.0	20.0	139	8.2	27.5	48	12.7	42.5	29	
Eschenbach 1553	5x/140, 20D, Illum	be hi		55	13.2	22.2	3.9	6.3	24.7	139	8.2	32.2	45	12.1	47.2	27	
Schweizer 192	5x-16D illum modular	be h	tilt	60	13.6	13.1	2.8	5.7	15.6	136	8.3	23.1	50	13.8	38.1	33	
Schweizer 193	4x, 12D, modular	be h		70	11.8	15.5	2.8	6.4	18.0	178	9.0	25.5	63	14.3	40.5	40	
COIL 6259	Rayliite 12 11.7D/3.9x	be ih		58	11.4	27.9	4.2	7.3	30.4	168	9.0	37.9	52	12.6	52.9	29	
Schweizer 193	4x-12D illum modular	be h	tilt	70	11.2	16.6	2.8	6.7	19.1	189	9.4	26.6	66	14.7	41.6	41	
COIL 5269	3.7x-11D Raylite 28	be ih		64	10.9	12.4	2.4	6.3	14.9	162	9.5	22.4	61	15.9	37.4	41	10.0cm-10D

Magnifiers ranked according to the resolution advantage (by EVD) they give when the eye is a moderate (10 cm) distance from the lens.

Equivalent Viewing Distances and eye-to-image distances (ey/im) are calculated for eye-lens distances of 2.5, 10 and 25 cm. (EVD = Eye-to-image dist / ER)

Each double ruled divider represents one line of visual acuity assuming size progression ratio = 5/4 .

Equivalent Viewing Power(EVP) and Equivalent Viewing Distance (EVD) conversion benchmarks are shown on the right at each horizontal divider.

Field sizes (fld) in millimeters are based on thin lens and small pupil assumptions. Field may be limited further by aberrations or by base of stand.

Illumination codes:- b = battery, r = rechargeable, e = electrical, i = incandescent, h = halogen (or xenon), f = fluorescent

For magnifiers with adjustable focus, listed specifications are for minimal image distance. For image at infinity, EVD = equiv focal length

TABLE 1   Illuminated Stand Magnifiers – Optical parameters

Manufacturer ID #	Descriptions	Illum code	Adjust	Lens size mm	Measured Fe D.	l' cm	ER x	z=2.5 EVD	ey/im	fld	z=10.0 EVD	ey/im	fld	z=25 EVD	ey/im	fld	EVD-EVI
Schweizer 21	4x-12D Leuchtlupe	be ih		69	9.3	19.5	2.8	7.8	22.0	217	10.5	29.5	73	15.8	44.5	44	
Schweizer 152/152H	3.5x illum	be ih		60	9.0	9.5	1.9	6.5	12.0	155	10.5	19.5	63	18.6	34.5	45	
Schweizer 196	3x, 8D, modular	be h		100 75	8.7	17.6	2.5	7.9	20.1	317	10.9	27.6	109	16.8	42.6	67	
Eschenbach 1555-1/204/3	3x-8D illum	be ih		80	7.6	7.0	1.5	6.2	9.5	198	11.1	17.0	89	20.9	32.0	67	
Eschenbach 1555	2.5x/250, Illum, angled	be hi		76	7.3	7.2	1.5	6.4	9.7	194	11.3	17.2	86	21.1	32.2	64	
Schweizer 22	3.5x-10D Leuchtlupe	b h		69	8.1	16.0	2.3	8.0	18.5	223	11.3	26.0	78	17.8	41.0	49	
Schweizer 1577	Leuchtlupe	b ih		55	7.7	10.9	1.8	7.3	13.4	161	11.3	20.9	63	19.5	35.9	43	
Schweizer 194	3x, 8D, modular	be h		85	7.9	16.5	2.3	8.2	19.0	280	11.5	26.5	98	18.0	41.5	61	
Schweizer 160	3.5x-10D flashlight mag	be ih		57	7.1	9.6	1.7	7.2	12.1	166	11.7	19.6	67	20.6	34.6	47	
Eschenbach 1580-1/204/3	3x-8D illum	be ih		100 50	7.6	16.8	2.3	8.5	19.3	338	11.7	26.8	117	18.3	41.8	73	
Eschenbach 1584-1/204/3	2.8x-7D illum	be ih		105	6.9	12.1	1.8	8.0	14.6	334	12.0	22.1	127	20.2	37.1	85	
Eschenbach 1588	3x-8D Vario SL illum	e	tilt	100 50	7.4	16.6	2.2	8.7	19.1	347	12.1	26.6	121	18.9	41.6	76	
Schweizer 153	2.5x-6D illum mag	be ih		98 46	7.5	11.7	1.8	7.9	14.2	311	12.1	21.7	119	20.5	36.7	80	
Eschenbach 1588	3x/250, variable illum	be hi	tilt	97 47	7.0	14.6	2.0	8.5	17.1	328	12.2	24.6	118	19.6	39.6	76	
Eschenbach 1580	3x/250, Illum	be hi	tilt	97 47	7.1	15.2	2.1	8.5	17.7	331	12.2	25.2	118	19.4	40.2	75	
Schweizer 154/154H	3x illum	be ih		100 75	6.8	12.9	1.9	8.2	15.4	328	12.2	22.9	122	20.2	37.9	81	
Eschenbach 1582-1/204/3	3x-8D illum	be ih		100 75	6.9	13.9	2.0	8.4	16.4	336	12.2	23.9	122	19.9	38.9	80	
Eschenbach 1584	2.8x/250, Illum	be hi	tilt	99 73	6.4	10.6	1.7	7.8	13.1	308	12.3	20.6	121	21.2	35.6	84	
Schweizer 196	3x-8D illum modular	be h	tilt	100 75	7.2	17.5	2.2	8.9	20.0	357	12.3	27.5	123	19.0	42.5	76	
Schweizer 194	3x-8D illum modular	be h	tilt	85	7.3	22.8	2.6	9.6	25.3	327	12.5	32.8	106	18.2	47.8	62	12.5cm-8D
Selsi 405 w/o reticle	10x illum	b i		22	28.5	10.1	1.6	7.9	12.6	70	12.7	20.1	28	22.2	35.1	20	
Eschenbach 1584	2.8x/250 illum stand mag	be i	tilt	98 74	6.2	14.5	1.9	8.9	17.0	350	12.9	24.5	126	20.8	39.5	47	
Selsi 406	5x illum	b i		47	14.7	13.9	1.9	8.8	16.4	166	12.9	23.9	61	21.0	38.9	39	
Schweizer 195	2.5x, 6D, modular	be h		100	5.8	16.1	1.9	9.6	18.6	384	13.5	26.1	135	21.2	41.1	85	
Eschenbach 1582	2.8x/250, Illum	be hi	tilt	98 73	5.1	13.8	1.7	9.6	16.3	376	14.0	23.8	137	22.8	38.8	90	
Schweizer 195	2.5x-6D illum modular	be h	tilt	100	5.6	17.5	2.0	10.2	20.0	408	14.0	27.5	140	21.7	42.5	87	16cm-16D
Selsi 405 c reticle	10x illum	b i		22	28.5	18.2	1.9	11.0	20.7	97	15.0	28.2	33	23.0	43.2	20	
B&L 81-34-80	1.5x illum	e i		100 50	4.4	24.2	2.1	12.9	26.7	515	16.5	34.2	165	23.8	49.2	95	20cm-5D

Magnifiers ranked according to the resolution advantage (by EVD) they give when the eye is a moderate (10 cm) distance from the lens.

Equivalent Viewing Distances and eye-to-image distances (ey/im) are calculated for eye-lens distances of 2.5, 10 and 25 cm. (EVD = Eye-to-image dist / ER)

Each double ruled divider represents one line of visual acuity assuming size progression ratio = 5/4 .

Equivalent Viewing Power(EVP) and Equivalent Viewing Distance (EVD) conversion benchmarks are shown on the right at each horizontal divider.

Field sizes (fld) in millimeters are based on thin lens and small pupil assumptions. Field may be limited further by aberrations or by base of stand.

Illumination codes:- b = battery,   r = rechargeable,   e = electrical,   i = incandescent,   h = halogen (or xenon),   f = fluorescent

For magnifiers with adjustable focus, listed specifications are for minimal image distance. For image at infinity, EVD = equiv focal length

TABLE 2 Non-Illuminated Stand Magnifiers – Optical parameters

Manufacturer ID #	Descriptions	Illum code	Adjust	Lens size (mm)	Fe (D)	l' (cm)	ER (x)	z=2.5 EVD	z=2.5 ey/im	z=2.5 fld	z=10.0 EVD	z=10.0 ey/im	z=10.0 fld	z=25 EVD	z=25 ey/im	z=25 fld	EVD-EV
Peak 8-16x a	8x-16x zoom		zoom	10	68.7	####	####	1.5	####	6	1.5	####	1	1.5	####	1	1.6cm-63D
COIL 4220 a	20x-76D Hi-power focusable		focus	26	53.6	####	####	1.9	####	19	1.9	####	5	1.9	####	2	
Peak 8-16x a'	8x-16x zoom		zoom	10	68.7	25.3	18.4	1.5	27.8	6	1.9	35.3	2	2.7	50.3	1	2.0cm-50D
COIL 4220 b	20x-76D Hi-power focusable		focus	26	53.6	13.4	8.2	1.9	15.9	20	2.9	23.4	7	4.7	38.4	5	
Peak 1964	22x stand			19	64.9	7.6	5.9	1.7	10.1	13	3.0	17.6	6	5.5	32.6	4	
Peak 8-16x b	8x-16x zoom		zoom	10	33.4	####	####	3.0	####	12	3.0	####	3	3.0	####	1	
Peak 1962	15x stand			19	45.3	18.4	9.3	2.2	20.9	17	3.0	28.4	6	4.7	43.4	4	
Schweizer 2618	10x Standlupe			28	38.1	37.4	15.3	2.6	39.9	29	3.1	47.4	9	4.1	62.4	5	3.2cm-32D
COIL 4215 a	15x-56D Hi-power focusable		focus	29	40.3	15.6	7.3	2.5	18.1	29	3.5	25.6	10	5.6	40.6	6	
COIL 4210	10x-36D Hi-power			36	30.7	38.0	12.7	3.2	40.5	46	3.8	48.0	14	5.0	63.0	7	
Peak 8-16x b'	8x-16x zoom		zoom	10	33.4	21.5	8.2	2.9	24.0	12	3.9	31.5	4	5.7	46.5	2	
Walters 109-104	4x, Horizon, scale		focus	29	32.5	22.4	8.3	3.0	24.9	35	3.9	32.4	11	5.7	47.4	7	
Eschenbach 1153	8x stand aplanatic			25	28.9	42.0	13.1	3.4	44.5	34	4.0	52.0	10	5.1	67.0	5	4.0cm-25D
COIL 4215 b	15x-56D Hi-power focusable		focus	29	40.3	8.2	4.3	2.5	10.7	29	4.2	18.2	12	7.7	33.2	9	
Peak 1961	10x stand			24	29.2	20.8	7.1	3.3	23.3	32	4.4	30.8	10	6.5	45.8	6	
Agfa 8x	8x lupe			24	29.2	20.7	7.0	3.3	23.2	32	4.4	30.7	10	6.5	45.7	6	
Agfa 8x	8x lupe			24	29.2	20.7	7.0	3.3	23.2	32	4.4	30.7	10	6.5	45.7	6	
Peak 2018	8x stand			23	26.0	30.3	8.9	3.7	32.8	34	4.5	40.3	10	6.2	55.3	6	
COIL 4208	8x-28D Hi-power			44	23.4	70.5	17.5	4.2	73.0	74	4.6	80.5	20	5.5	95.5	10	
Walters 109-108	8x, Horizon,		focus	27	25.8	26.0	7.7	3.7	28.5	40	4.7	36.0	13	6.6	51.0	7	
Selsi 404	Chrome paperweight			60	15.3	4.0	2.9	2.2	6.5	54	4.8	14.0	29	10.1	29.0	24	
Eschenbach 2624	8x stand mag			30	23.3	28.0	7.5	4.0	30.5	49	5.0	38.0	15	7.0	53.0	8	5.0cm-20D
COIL 5123	8x-28D Hi-power			36	23.5	24.5	6.7	4.0	27.0	58	5.1	34.5	18	7.3	49.5	11	
Eschenbach 2624	8x stand			35	23.5	20.6	5.8	4.0	23.1	55	5.2	30.6	18	7.8	45.6	11	
Walters 109-008	8x angled table mag			22	19.9	35.4	8.1	4.7	37.9	41	5.6	45.4	12	7.5	60.4	7	
COIL 4206	6x-20D Hi-power			44	18.7	49.1	10.2	5.1	51.6	89	5.8	59.1	26	7.3	74.1	13	
B&L 81-31-02	5x aspheric stand mag			48	17.6	30.9	6.5	5.2	33.4	100	6.3	40.9	31	8.7	55.9	17	6.3cm-16D
Eschenbach 2626	6x stand			50	16.9	14.0	3.4	4.9	16.5	98	7.1	24.0	36	11.6	39.0	23	
COIL 5428	6x-20D large cataract			47	16.9	13.5	3.3	4.9	16.0	92	7.2	23.5	34	11.8	38.5	22	
B&L 81-31-03	4x aspheric stand mag			48	16.4	15.0	3.5	5.1	17.5	98	7.2	25.0	35	11.5	40.0	22	
Walters 8042	10x, Horizon		focus	23	15.0	27.1	5.1	5.8	29.6	54	7.3	37.1	17	10.3	52.1	9	
Eschenbach 2626	6x stand mag			47	15.7	14.5	3.3	5.2	17.0	98	7.5	24.5	35	12.1	39.5	23	
Selsi 402	Jupiter 4x			59	14.3	18.6	3.7	5.8	21.1	136	7.8	28.6	46	11.9	43.6	28	
Schweizer 320/40	24D visolett			40	23.2	2.5	1.6	3.2	5.0	51	7.9	12.5	32	17.4	27.5	28	
Eschenbach 1411	bright field paperweight			40	22.9	2.6	1.6	3.2	5.1	51	7.9	12.6	32	17.4	27.6	28	
Eschenbach 2050	3.5x hand held/stand/pocket		folds	60	13.8	20.8	3.9	6.0	23.3	144	8.0	30.8	48	11.8	45.8	28	8cm-12.5D
COIL 5850	Bright Magnifier			50	20.4	3.1	1.6	3.5	5.6	70	8.1	13.1	41	17.5	28.1	35	
Eschenbach 1421	Bright field Mag			62	17.2	4.6	1.8	4.0	7.1	99	8.2	14.6	51	16.5	29.6	41	
Eschenbach 2627	4x stand			60	13.3	19.8	3.6	6.1	22.3	147	8.2	29.8	49	12.3	44.8	30	
Schweizer 2616	4x Standlupe			55	13.3	19.9	3.6	6.2	22.4	135	8.2	29.9	45	12.3	44.9	27	
Schweizer 320/65	16D visolett			65	15.6	5.1	1.8	4.2	7.6	110	8.4	15.1	56	16.8	30.1	44	
Selsi 403	Dome			53	16.5	4.0	1.7	3.9	6.5	83	8.4	14.0	45	17.4	29.0	37	
Eschenbach 1420	bright field paperweight			65	15.6	4.6	1.7	4.1	7.1	107	8.5	14.6	55	17.3	29.6	45	
Walters 109-005	5x angled table mag			24	12.2	41.3	6.0	7.3	43.8	70	8.5	51.3	21	11.0	66.3	11	
Schweizer 322	4x stand mag			55	12.5	20.1	3.5	6.4	22.6	142	8.6	30.1	47	12.9	45.1	28	
Schweizer 320/55	16D visolett			55	16.0	3.7	1.6	3.9	6.2	86	8.6	13.7	47	18.0	28.7	40	
Eschenbach 1425	bright field paperweight			65 32	15.2	4.3	1.7	4.1	6.8	107	8.7	14.3	56	17.7	29.3	46	
Schweizer 321	4x stand mag			55	11.4	19.2	3.2	6.8	21.7	150	9.1	29.2	50	13.8	44.2	30	
COIL 5214 b	4x-12D Hi-power		tiltb	80	10.8	69.3	8.5	8.5	71.8	270	9.3	79.3	75	11.1	94.3	36	
COIL 5214 a	4x-12D Hi-power		tilt a	80	10.8	67.0	8.2	8.4	69.5	270	9.3	77.0	75	11.2	92.0	36	
Eschenbach 2625	4x-12D stand mag			63 53	10.5	13.3	2.4	6.6	15.8	162	9.7	23.3	61	15.9	38.3	40	
Schweizer 320/90	12D visolett			90	10.8	6.9	1.7	5.4	9.4	194	9.7	16.9	87	18.3	31.9	66	
Eschenbach 1430	bright field paperweight			90	10.7	6.6	1.7	5.3	9.1	192	9.7	16.6	88	18.6	31.6	67	
Eschenbach 2625	4x stand			70 55	10.1	12.2	2.2	6.6	14.7	184	10.0	22.2	70	16.7	37.2	47	10cm-10D
COIL 5474	3.7x-11D stand			64 52	8.8	18.5	2.4	8.0	21.0	204	10.8	28.5	69	16.5	43.5	42	
Walters 109-002,R-324	3x table mag			74	7.8	8.2	1.6	6.5	10.7	193	11.1	18.2	82	20.2	33.2	60	
Walters 109-010	10x table		focus	24	30.7	9.9	1.7	7.1	12.4	68	11.4	19.9	27	20.0	34.9	19	
Eschenbach 2623	3x-8D stand mag			93 72	7.7	16.8	2.3	8.4	19.3	313	11.6	26.8	109	18.2	41.8	68	
COIL 5213 a	3x-8D Hi power		tilt a	81	7.9	22.4	2.8	9.0	24.9	291	11.7	47.4	55	17.1	47.4	55	
COIL 5213 b	3x-8D Hi power		tilt b	81	7.9	22.9	2.8	9.0	25.4	293	11.7	32.9	95	17.1	47.9	55	
COIL 5472	3x-8D large stand			94 69	6.9	14.1	2.0	8.4	16.6	316	12.2	24.1	115	19.8	39.1	74	12.5cm-8D
Donegan A-2072	2x rectangular stand			97 49	6.5	14.6	2.0	8.8	17.1	339	12.6	24.6	122	20.3	39.6	78	
Eschenbach 2623	8x stand			100 75	6.5	15.5	2.0	9.0	18.0	359	12.7	25.5	127	20.2	40.5	81	
Eschenbach 2622	3x stand			100 75	6.3	21.0	2.3	10.1	23.5	403	13.3	31.0	133	19.7	46.0	79	16.0cm-6.3D
COIL 5855	1.78x-3D stand			140 100	1.9	26.5	1.5	19.1	29.0	###	24.1	36.5	337	34.0	51.5	190	25cm-4D
Selsi 433a	8x Waltex		focus	24	27.9	32.6	1.6	22.0	35.1	212	26.8	42.6	64	36.2	57.6	35	32cm-3.2D
Selsi 433b	8x Waltex		focus	24	27.9	74.8	1.8	43.1	77.3	413	47.2	84.8	113	55.6	99.8	53	50cm-2D

Magnifiers ranked according to the resolution advantage (by EVD) they give when the eye is a moderate (10 cm) distance from the lens.

Equivalent Viewing Distances and eye-to-image distances (ey/im) are calculated for eye-lens distances of 2.5, 10 and 25 cm. (EVD = Eye-to-image dist / ER)

Each double ruled divider represents one line of visual acuity assuming size progression ratio = 5/4 .

Equivalent Viewing Power(EVP) and Equivalent Viewing Distance (EVD) conversion benchmarks are shown on the right at each horizontal divider.

Field sizes (fld) in millimeters are based on thin lens and small pupil assumptions. Field may be limited further by aberrations or by base of stand.

Illumination codes:- b = battery, r = rechargeable, e = electrical, i = incandescent, h = halogen (or xenon), f = fluorescent

For magnifiers with adjustable focus, listed specifications are for minimal image distance. For image at infinity, EVD = equiv focal length

Appendix C: The Equivalent Viewing System of Magnification Rating

Table 3   Hand Held Magnifiers - Optical Parameters

Manufacturer ID #	Ratings	Descriptions	Illum code	Lens size mm	EVD cm	Fe D	EVD-EVP
Eschenbach #1510-1004.1	10X 36 D	Illuminated Pocket	b i	35	2.7	36.7	3.2cm-32D
B&L #81-23-63-1	7X 28 D	Lenses together 7x		37	3.9	25.4	4.0cm-25D
Magna-lite #300	6X 24 D	Illuminated mag	b i	30 -30	4.3	23.4	
Eschenbach #1510-704	7X 24 D	Illuminated Pocket	b i	35	4.3	23.2	
Eschenbach 2655 50	6X 20 D	6x/100 round		50	4.5	22.3	
B&L #81-33-86-2	6X 24 D	Bifocal inset lens		22	4.9	20.6	
B&L #81-33-76-2	6X 24 D	Bifocal inset lens		22	4.9	20.3	
B&L #81-41-37	5X 20 D	5x clip-on		24	5.0	20.1	5.0cm-20D
B&L #81-31-33	5X 20 D	5x Packette		35	5.3	18.8	
Eschenbach #1510-1004.2	5X 16 D	Bifocal		25	5.3	18.8	
Eschenbach #2655 60	5X 16 D	5x/140 round		60	5.3	18.8	
Eschenbach #1510-504	5X 16 D	Illuminated Pocket	b i	58	5.4	18.6	
COIL #5206	6X 20 D	Hi Power		50	5.5	18.0	
B&L #81-31-22	5X 20 D	5x round hand		50	5.6	17.9	
COIL #5460	6X 20 D	Cataract Hand Reader		47	5.6	17.8	
Eschenbach #1571	6X 20 D	Illuminated Pocket	b i	30	5.7	17.6	
Eschenbach #2650 50	6X 20 D	6x round		50	5.8	17.2	
B&L #81-41-78	4X 16 D	Objective lens		24	6.1	16.4	
B&L #81-41-78	3X 12 D	Eyelens 3/4/7x clip		24	6.3	16.0	
B&L #81-23-63-2	4X 16 D	LENS#1 4X		37	6.3	15.9	6.3cm-16D
Eschenbach #1510-404	4X 12 D	Illuminated Pocket	b i	35	6.4	15.7	
B&L #81-23-54	4X 16 D	4x folding pocket		37	6.4	15.5	
COIL #5798	4.8X 15 D	LVA		50	6.7	14.9	
Eschenbach #2655 70	4X 12 D	4x/180 round		70	6.8	14.7	
Eschenbach #2050	3.5X 10 D	h-held/stand/pocket		60	7.3	13.8	
Eschenbach #1572	4X 12 D	Illuminated pocket	b i	60	7.2	13.8	
COIL #5844.2	4.25X 13 D	Bifocal		35	7.8	12.8	8.0cm-12.5D
B&L #81-33-52	3.5X 14 D	3.5x Mini-lite	b i	32 -32	8.1	12.3	
Magna-lite #100	3X 12 D	Illuminated mag	b i	30 -30	8.2	12.2	
COIL #5247	4.42X 13.7 D	Windsor		48	8.2	12.2	
B&L #81-23-63-3	3X 12 D	Lens#2 3x		37	9.1	11.0	
B&L #81-23-32	3X 12 D	3x Packette		37	9.2	10.8	
COIL #5204	4X 12 D	Hi Power		80	9.5	10.5	
Eschenbach #2660	4X 12 D	4x rectangular		70 -55	9.9	10.1	10.0cm-10D
Eschenbach #1740-160	3.5X 10 D	Folding Pocket		60	10.2	9.8	
Eschenbach #2655 750	3.5X 10 D	3.5x/250 rectangular		75 -50	10.6	9.5	
Eschenbach #1510-305	3.5X 10 D	Illuminated Pocket	b i	75 -50	10.8	9.3	
COIL #5432	3.7X 11 D	Minor Rectangular		64 -52	10.9	9.1	
COIL #5285	3.4X 9.5 D	Oro		50	11.2	8.9	
B&L #81-26-05	2X 8 D	2x attached case		50	12.5	8.0	12.5cm-8D
Eschenbach #2655 150	3X 8 D	3x/250 rectangular		100 -50	12.8	7.8	
COIL #5203	3X 8 D	Hi Power		81	13.2	7.6	
COIL #5442	3.3X 8 D	Large Rectangular		94 -69	14.0	7.1	
Eschenbach 2655 175	2.75X 7 D	2.75/250 rectangular		100 -75	14.6	6.9	
Eschenbach #1575	3X 8 D	Illuminated Pocket	b i	75 -50	15.1	6.6	16cm-6.3D
COIL #5248	2.6X 6.4 D	Windsor		70 -50	16.5	6.1	
COIL #5438	2.62X 6.5 D	Minor Rectangular		83 -64	16.6	6.0	
COIL #5449	2.5X 6 D	Major Rectangular		102 -75	17.2	5.8	
Eschenbach #1573	2.5X 6 D	Illuminated Pocket	b i	80	18.6	5.4	
COIL #5249	2.3X 5.3 D	Windsor		98	19.2	5.2	
B&L #81-90-08	2X 8 D	rectractable illum	b i	50 -50	19.8	5.1	
COIL #5178	2.3X 5.3 D	Easi Twin main lens		105	19.5	5.1	
COIL #5216	2.3X 5.2 D	Hi Power		96 -71	19.9	5.0	20cm-5D
Luxo 5D lens	5 D	Luxo +5	e f	71	20.7	4.8	
B&L #81-33-86-1	2X 8 D	Rectangular illuminated mag	e i	100 -50	21.5	4.7	
B&L #81-33-76-1	2X 8 D	Main lens Rect		100 -50	21.7	4.6	25cm-4.0D
Big Eye Lens Big eye	2X 4 D	Big eye	e i	120	31.2	3.2	32cm-3.2D
COIL #5215	1.7X 2.8 D	Hi Power		96 -71	36.5	2.7	
B&L #81-33-90	2X 8 D	Magna-viewer		125 -100	40.5	2.5	40cm-2.5D
B&L #81-90-07	2X 8 D	Magna-page		180 -260	41.4	2.4	
COIL #5844.1	1.7X 3 D	Flexi-Mag		140 -100	44.5	2.2	
COIL #5820	1.7X 3 D	Easi-View Hands-Free		145 -105	44.6	2.2	50cm-2D

Magnifiers ranked by EVD which indicates the resolution advantage obtained when the lens is used to give an image at infinity.

When a hand held magnifier is remote (one focal length or greater) from the eye, the distance Rx should be used to obtain best resolution.

When a hand held magnifier is held close to the eye, resolution may be increased by using a reading addition or accommodation.

Each double ruled divider represents one line of visual acuity, assuming the size progression ratio = 5/4 .

Equivalent Viewing Distance (EVD) and Equivalent Viewing Power(EVP) benchmarks are shown at each horizontal divider.

Illumination codes:- b = battery,   r = rechargeable,   e = electrical,   i = incandescent,   h = halogen (or xenon),   f = fluorescent

TABLE 4 Prism Readers - Optical Parameters

IDENTIFICATION			FRAME				POWER		CONVERGENCE DIST.		PHYSICAL	
Manufacturer	Power (D.)	Prism Δ	Frame		Eye Size (mm)	DBL (mm)	Equiv Pwr (D.)	eq focal l (cm.)	For PD = 58 (cm.)	For PD = 68 (cm.)	thickness (mm)	weight (g.)
Mattingly	4.00	6	DeepSee	HE	45	22.5	3.75	26.4	37.6	44.5	7.1	32
Mattingly	5.00	7	DeepSee	HE	45	22.5	4.63	21.2	29.9	35.5	8.5	33
Mattingly	6.00	8	DeepSee	HE	45	22.5	5.50	18.0	23.2	27.6	9.6	37
Mattingly	7.00	9	DeepSee	HE	45	22.5	6.38	15.6	19.9	23.8	11.2	39
Mattingly	8.00	10	DeepSee	HE	45	22.5	7.38	13.5	15.3	18.4	11.9	41
Mattingly	10.00	12	DeepSee	HE	45	22.5	9.13	11.0	10.9	13.3	12.9	43
Mattingly	12.00	14	DeepSee	HE	45	22.5	10.63	9.4	8.7	10.7	15.8	47
Mattingly	4.00	6	DeepSee	HE	49	23.5	3.75	26.4	33.4	39.6	8.8	40
Mattingly	5.00	7	DeepSee	HE	49	23.5	4.63	21.2	27.5	32.8	9.8	43
Mattingly	6.00	8	DeepSee	HE	49	23.5	5.50	17.9	19.9	23.8	10.9	44
Mattingly	7.00	9	DeepSee	HE	49	23.5	6.38	15.4	18.0	21.6	13.0	49
Mattingly	8.00	10	DeepSee	HE	49	23.5	7.25	13.6	14.8	17.8	13.7	50
Mattingly	10.00	12	DeepSee	HE	49	23.5	9.00	11.1	10.6	12.9	16.0	56
Mattingly	12.00	14	DeepSee	HE	49	23.5	10.50	9.5	8.5	10.5	18.1	62
Mattingly	6.00	8	Thin	HE	45	22.5	5.75	17.1	29.2	34.7	10.6	32
Mattingly	8.00	10	Thin	HE	45	22.5	7.63	13.0	21.2	25.4	10.1	33
Mattingly	10.00	12	Thin	HE	45	22.5	9.38	10.6	15.9	19.1	13.2	34
Mattingly	12.00	14	Thin	HE	45	22.5	10.75	9.3	13.0	15.7	13.2	36
Mattingly	6.00	8	Thin	HE	49	23.5	5.88	17.0	25.9	30.8	9.0	34
Mattingly	8.00	10	Thin	HE	49	23.5	7.63	13.0	19.1	22.9	10.6	37
Mattingly	10.00	12	Thin	HE	49	23.5	9.38	10.6	14.4	17.4	13.3	39
Mattingly	12.00	14	Thin	HE	49	23.5	12.50	8.0	11.2	13.6	12.0	40

Appendix D:
Selected Readings From
Low Vision—The Reference

Gregory L. Goodrich

Low Vision—The Reference is a comprehensive list of low vision related publications that is published and updated annually by The Lighthouse, Inc., New York, New York. It is available in both print and electronic (DOS and Macintosh) versions.

These references are listed according to date of publication for the convenience of the reader. They represent a small number of the excellent publications related to low vision available in the more comprehensive text.

LOW VISION DEVICES

Cole RG. A Functional Approach to the Optics of Low Vision Devices. In RG Cole, BP Rosenthal (eds), Remediation and Management of Low Vision. St. Louis: Mosby–Year Book, 1996;139.

Goodrich GL, Sacco T. Visual Function with High-Tech Low Vision Devices. In RG Cole, BP Rosenthal (eds), Remediation and Management of Low Vision. St. Louis: Mosby–Year Book, 1996;197.

Rosenthal BP, Hoeft WW. A Functional Approach to the Fitting of Spectacle-Mounted Telescopic Systems. In RG Cole, BP Rosenthal (eds), Remediation and Management of Low Vision. St. Louis: Mosby–Year Book, 1996;267.

Williams DR. Functional Adaptive Devices. In RG Cole, BP Rosenthal (eds), Remediation and Management of Low Vision. St. Louis: Mosby–Year Book, 1996;71.

Reich LN. Field of view and equivalent viewing power of near-vision telescopes. Optom Vis Sci 1995;72:411.

Spitzberg LA, Goodrich GL. New ergonomic stand magnifiers. J Am Optom Assoc 1995;66:25.

Bailey IL, Bullimore MA, Greer RB, Mattingly WB. Low vision magnifiers—their optical parameters and methods for prescribing. Optom Vis Sci 1994;71:689.

Brabyn J, Colenbrander A, Winderl M. Improving the ergonomics of popular low vision telescopes. J Vis Rehabil 1994;8:12.

Gurwood AS, Brilliant R. Basic optics of telescopes: a review. J Vis Rehabil 1994;8:3.

Keswick C. Field Enhancing Devices. In G Clarke, T Heyes (eds), Visions in Mobility: Proceedings of the International Mobility Conference 7. Kew, Australia: Royal Guide Dogs Associations of Australia, 1994;233.

Spitzberg LA, Chen S. The design of a zoom stand magnifier—a new low vision device. Optom Vis Sci 1994;71:613.

Spitzberg LA, Goodrich GL. New Ergonomic Stand Magnifiers. In AC Kooijman, PL Looijestijn, JA Welling, GJ van der Wildt (eds), Low Vision: Research and New Developments in Rehabilitation. Amsterdam: International Optical Society Press, 1994;159.

Spitzberg LA, Goodrich GL, Perez-Franco AM. Reading and Vertical Magnification with Retinitis Pigmentosa. In AC Kooijman, PL Looijestijn, JA Welling, GJ van der Wildt (eds), Low Vision: Research and New Developments in Rehabilitation. Amsterdam: International Optical Society Press, 1994;275.

Spitzberg LA, Ming Q. Depth of field of plus lenses and reading telescopes. Optom Vis Sci 1994;71:115.

Fraser KE. Child with telescopic lens prescription. J Vis Rehabil 1993;7:5.

Greene HA, Pekar J, Brilliant R, et al. Use of spectacle mounted telescope systems by the visually impaired. J Am Optom Assoc 1993;64:507.

Jose R. Fit-over sunfilters. J Vis Rehabil 1993;7:15.

Nguyen A, Nguyen A-T, Hemenger RP, Williams DR. Resolution, field of view, and retinal illuminance of miniaturized bioptic telescopes and their clinical significance. J Vis Rehabil 1993;7:5.

Perez AM. New bifocal option: UniVision by Unilens. J Vis Rehabil 1993;7:15.

Porter FI, Goldberg J, White JM, Koval AV. Role of clinical factors in the outcome of low vision rehabilitation with telescopic spectacles. Clin Vis Sci 1993;8:473.

Ray JS. Prescribing high addition bifocals for low-vision patients with specific functional needs. J Vis Rehabil 1993;7:6.

Rosenbloom AA, Morgan MW (eds). Vision and Aging: General and Clinical Perspectives (2nd ed). Boston: Butterworth–Heinemann, 1993.

Stelmack J, Guggenheim M, Carman-Merrifield C. Patient evaluation of the 7x30 Beecher Mirage low vision system. J Vis Impair Blind 1993;87:408.

Temel A, Bavbeck T, Kanpolat A. Clinical application of contact lens telescopes. Int J Rehabil Res 1993;16:148.

Wuebolt GE, Patel BC, Silver JH, Collin JR. Brow-supported spectacle frames for nasal bridge reconstruction and other deformities. Arch Ophthalmol 1993;111:162.

Bolduc M, Simonet P, Gresset J, Melillo M. To use or not to use the refractive correction along with hand-held magnifiers. Optom Vis Sci 1992;69:769.

Brabyn J. Problems to be overcome in high-tech devices for the visually impaired. Optom Vis Sci 1992;69:42.

Cole RG. The four diopter intermediate. J Vis Rehabil 1992;6:13.

Edmonds SA. Contact Lens Consideration for Low Vision Management. In RG Cole, BP Rosenthal (eds), Problems in Optometry: Patient and Practice Management in Low Vision (vol 4). Philadelphia: Lippincott, 1994.

Freeman PB. Clinical evaluation of the Clear Image II lens. J Vis Rehabil 1992;6:5.

Freeman PB. Posture and the use of near low vision devices. J Vis Rehabil 1992;6:1.

Greene HA, Beadles R, Pekar J. Challenges in applying autofocus technology to low vision telescopes. Optom Vis Sci 1992;69:25.

Hoeft WW. The Amorphic Lens. In RG Cole, BP Rosenthal (eds), Problems in Optometry: Patient and Practice Management in Low Vision (vol 4). Philadelphia: Lippincott, 1992.

Lowe J, Drasdo N. Using a binocular field expander on a wide-field search task. Optom Vis Sci 1992;69:186.

Massof RW, Rickman DL. Obstacles encountered in the development of the low vision enhancement system. Optom Vis Sci 1992;69:32.

Moss GS. Consideration on dispensing low vision devices. J Vis Impair Blind 1992;86:88.

Porter FI, White JM, Goldberg J, et al. Predicting successful low vision rehabilitation with telescopic spectacles. J Vis Impair Blind 1992;86:29.

Porter TI. A loaner system for more complex low vision devices. J Vis Rehabil 1992;6:13.

Rieger G. Improvement of contrast sensitivity with yellow filter glasses. Can J Ophthalmol 1992;27:137.

Yaniglos SS, Leigh RJ. Refinement of an optical device that stabilizes vision in patients with nystagmus. Optom Vis Sci 1992;69:447.

Barron C. Bioptic telescopic spectacles for motor vehicle driving. J Am Optom Assoc 1991;62:37.

Cohen JM, Waiss B. Comparison of reading speed in normal observers through different forms of equivalent power low vision devices. Optom Vis Sci 1991;68:127.

Cole RG. Considerations in Low Vision Prescribing. In BP Rosenthal, RG Cole (eds), Problems in Optometry: A Structured Approach to Low Vision Care (vol 3). Philadelphia: Lippincott, 1991.

Finkelstein D, Feinberg SJ, Flom RE, et al. Visual prostheses and visual rehabilitation in low vision. Curr Opin Ophthalmol 1991;2:729.

Fonda GE. Designing half-eye binocular spectacle magnifiers. Surv Ophthalmol 1991;36:149.

Fryer A, Leat SJ, Rumney NJ. Do low vision aids end up in the drawer? Ophthalmic Physiol Optics 1991;11:398.

Goodrich GL. Computer Technology for the Blind and Partially Sighted in the United States: Does Legislation Have an Impact? In PL Emiliani, A Parreno (eds), Access to Computer Systems by Blind Persons. London: Royal National Institute for the Blind, 1991.

Greene HA. The Ocutech Vision Enhancing System (VES): A New Low Vision Spectacle. In BP Rosenthal, RG Cole (eds), Problems in Optometry: A Structured Approach to Low Vision Care (vol 3). Philadelphia: Lippincott, 1991.

Greene HA, Pekar J, Brilliant R, et al. The Ocutech Vision Enhancing System (VES): utilization and preference study. J Am Optom Assoc 1991;62:19.

Harkins T, Maino JH. The BITA telescope: a first impression. J Am Optom Assoc 1991;62:28.

Hoeft WW. The Microspiral Galilean Telescope. In BP Rosenthal, RG Cole (eds), Problems in Optometry: A Structured Approach to Low Vision Care (vol 3). Philadelphia: Lippincott, 1991.

Innes A. Prescribing Spectacles for Low Vision Patients. In BP Rosenthal, RG Cole (eds), Problems in Optometry: A Structured Approach to Low Vision Care (vol 3). Philadelphia: Lippincott, 1991.

Peli E, Goldstein R, Young G, et al. Image enhancement for the visually impaired: simulation and experimental results. Invest Ophthalmol Vis Sci 1991;32:2337.

Reich LN. Adjustable focus telescopes for near vision. Optom Vis Sci 1991;68:183.

Rosenthal B. A short history on the development of low vision aids. J Vis Rehabil 1991;5:1.

Spitzberg LA. A patient's experience on driving with a bioptic. J Vis Rehabil 1991;5:17.

Spitzberg LA, Jose RT. An improved fitting position for the new Behind-the-Lens (BTL) telescope. J Vis Rehabil 1991;5:5.

Spitzberg LA, Jose RT, Kuether CL. Behind-the-Lens Telescope. In BP Rosenthal, RG Cole (eds), Problems in Optometry: A Structured Approach to Low Vision Care (vol 3). Philadelphia: Lippincott, 1991.

Waiss B, Cohen JM. Modification of common low vision devices for uncommon needs. J Am Optom Assoc 1991;62:65.

Walls MK, Molenda MM. Training procedures for more cosmetically appealing miniaturized telescopes. J Vis Rehabil 1991;5:11.

Wilkins A, Neary C. Some visual, optometric and perceptual effects of coloured glasses. Ophthalmic Physiol Opt 1991;11:163.

Williams DR. The Bi-Level Telemicroscopic Apparatus (BITA). In BP Rosenthal, RG Cole (eds), Problems in Optometry: A Structured Approach to Low Vision Care (vol 3). Philadelphia: Lippincott, 1991.

Williams DR. An evaluation of the optical characteristics of prismatic half-eye spectacles for the low vision patient. J Vis Rehabil 1991;5:21.

Buser F. High Quality Low Technology in Low Vision. In AW Johnston, M Lawrence (eds), Low Vision Ahead II Conference Proceedings. Kooyong, Australia: Association for the Blind, 1990.

Chung STL, Johnston AW. New stand magnifiers do not meet rated levels of performance. Clin Exp Optom 1990;73:194.

Gustafsson J, Polland W. Multifocal Head-Borne High-Power Glasses: A New Design for Reading Aids. In AW Johnston, M Lawrence (eds), Low Vision Ahead II Conference Proceedings. Kooyong, Australia: Association for the Blind, 1990.

Johnston AW. A Decision Path for the Prescription of Low Vision Aids. In AW Johnston, M Lawrence (eds), Low Vision Ahead II Conference Proceedings. Kooyong, Australia: Association for the Blind, 1990.

Lindstrom JI. Technological solutions for visually impaired people in Sweden. J Vis Impair Blind 1990;84:513.

Otto D, Woo GC. Notes on the use of low magnification telescopes in low vision care. Clin Exp Optom 1990;73:37.

Robinson J, Story S, Kuyk T. Evaluation of two night-vision devices. J Vis Impair Blind 1990;84:539.

Shull LE, Kuyk T. Wide angle mobility light (WAML) follow-up. J Vis Impair Blind 1990;84:78.

Siwoff RS. Patient preference between new cosmetically appealing spectacle telescope systems. J Vis Rehabil 1990;4:7.

Strong G, Bevers P. Non-Generic Considerations When Prescribing High Technology Sight Enhancement Systems. In AW Johnston, M Lawrence (eds), Low Vision Ahead II Conference Proceedings. Kooyong, Australia: Association for the Blind, 1990.

Taylor DG. Telescopic spectacles for driving: user data satisfaction, preferences and effects in vocational, educational and personal tasks: a study in Illinois. J Vis Rehabil 1990;4:29

Zigman S. Vision enhancement using a short wavelength light-absorbing filter. Optom Vis Sci 1990;67:100.

Campbell MCW, Ellison PJ, Strong JG, Lovasik IV. Unexpectedly large enhancement of a severely constricted field with reverse Galilean telescopes. Optom Vis Sci 1989;66:276.

Eldred KB. Use of a contact lens as a microscope. J Vis Rehabil 1989;3:23.

Herget M, Williams A. New aids for low vision diabetics. Am J Nurs 1989;89:1319.

Jampolski A, Brabyn J, Lewis A, Winder M. Two experimental low vision illumination aids. J Vis Rehabil 1989;3:33.

Jose RT, Spitzberg LA, Kuether CL. A behind the lens reversed (BTLR) telescope. J Vis Rehabil 1989;3:37.

Lawton TB. Improved reading performance using individualized compensation filters for observers with losses in central vision. Ophthalmology (Rochester) 1989;96:115.

Loshin OS, Juday RD. The programmable remapper: clinical applications for patients with field defects. Optom Vis Sci 1989;66:389.

Spitzberg LA, Jose RT, Kuether CL. Behind the lens telescope: a new concept in bioptics. Optom Vis Sci 1989;66:616.

Watson G. Competencies and a bibliography addressing students' use of low vision devices. J Vis Impair Blind 1989;83:160.

Bailey IL. Determining the angle for bioptic telescopes. J Vis Rehabil 1988;2:5.

Cole RG. A unified approach to the optics of low vision aids. J Vis Rehabil 1988;2:23.

Goodrich GL. Driving and telescopic aids: a bibliography. J Vis Rehabil 1988;2:21.

Lippmann O, Corn AL, Lewis AC. Bioptic telescopic spectacles and driving performance: a study in Texas. J Vis Impair Blind 1988;82:182.

Nasrallah FP, Jalkh AE, Freidman GR, et al. Visual results with low-vision aids in age-related macular degeneration. Am J Ophthalmol 1988;106:730.

Schwartzenberg T, Merin S, Nawratzki I, Yanko L. Low-vision aids in Stargardt's disease. Ann Ophthalmol 1988;20:428.

Zahn JR, Favero B, Horgan J. Model of visual rehabilitation utilizing specialized optical technology. J Vis Impair Blind 1988;2:59.

Abadi RV, Papas EB. Visual performance with artificial iris contact lenses. J Br CL Assoc 1987;10:10.

Aoki S, Furuta N. The effects of absorptive lenses on low vision clients. Bull Tok Metropolitan Rehabil Center 1987;27.

Bailey IL. Prescribing Low Vision Aids. In GC Woo (ed), Low Vision: Principles and Application. New York: Springer, 1987.

Bailey IL. A critical view of ocular telephoto systems. CLAO J 1987;13:217.

Edmonds S, Edmonds SE. Prismatic scanning vs. standard microscope techniques. J Vis Rehabil 1987;1:49.

Greene HA, Pekar J. Bioptic telescope utilization survey. J Vis Rehabil 1987;1:39.

Katz M, Citek K, Price I. Optical properties of low vision telescopes. J Am Optom Assoc 1987;58:320.

Overbury O, Jackson WB, Hagenson C. Factors affecting the successful use of low vision aids. Can J Ophthalmol 1987;22:205.

Wheatley G. A follow-up study of optical low vision aid use and stressful life events. J Vis Rehabil 1987;1:53.

Woo GC. An Overview on the Use of a Low Vision Magnification Telescope in Low Vision. In GC Woo (ed), Low Vision: Principles and Applications. New York: Springer, 1987.

Byer A. Magnification limitations of a contact lens telescope. Am J Optom Physiol Optics 1986;63:724.

Campbell MCW, Ellison PJ, Strong JG. Investigation of optical factors in unexpectedly large field enhancements. Am J Optom Physiol Optics 1986;63:87.

Goodrich GL, Mehr EB. Eccentric viewing training and low vision aids: current practice and implications of peripheral retinal research. Am J Optom Physiol Optics 1986;63:119.

Greig DE, West ML, Overbury O. Successful use of low vision aids: visual and psychological factors. J Vis Impair Blind 1986;80:985.

Kjeldstad A, LaGrow SJ. The effect of binocular distance aids on localization rates of three visually impaired persons. Educ Vis Handicapped 1986;28:101.

Maino JH, McMahon TT. Noir filters in low vision. J Am Optom Assoc 1986;575:532.

Whittaker SG, Miller LR, Cummings RW, Miller-Shaffer H. Retinal image stabilization systems for patients with unsteady fixation. Invest Ophthalmol Vis Sci (Suppl) 1986;27:105.

Lauber H. Telescopic spectacles. Arch Ophthalmol 1915;89:401.

Scott K. Telescopic spectacles. Ophthalmology 1913;9:444.

Stoll KL. Telescopic spectacles: their history, practicability and future. Lancet 1912;108:120.

Scott K. Telescopic eyeglasses. Ophthalmology 1911;7:445.

von Rodgin M. Telescopic and microscopic spectacles. Archos Soc Am Oftal Optom 1910;2:237.

LOW VISION AND DRIVING

Higgins KE. Low Vision Driving Among Normally-Sighted Drivers. In RG Cole, BP Rosenthal (eds), Remediation and Management of Low Vision. St. Louis: Mosby–Year Book, 1996;225.

Politzer MR. Vision rehabilitation therapy for the bioptic driver. J Am Optom Assoc 1995;66:18.

Corn AL, Sacks SZ. The impact of non-driving on adults with visual impairments. J Vis Impair Blind 1994;88:53.

Goodrich GL. Status of low vision and driving. J Vis Rehabil 1994;8:9.

Jolly N, Callegari J. The Effect of Reduced Acuity on the Ability to See Road Signs. In C Clarke, T Heyes (eds), Visions in Mobility: Proceedings of the International Mobility Conference 7. Kew, Australia: Royal Guide Dogs Associations of Australia, 1994;349.

Wood JM, Troutbeck R. Effect of visual impairment on driving. Hum Factors 1994;36:476.

Szlyk JP, Brigell M, Seiple M. Effects of age and hemianopic visual field loss on driving. Optom Vis Sci 1993;70:1031.

Szlyk JP, Fishman GA, Severing K. Evaluation of driving performance in patients with juvenile macular dystrophies. Arch Ophthalmol 1993;111:207.

Bailey IL, Sheedy JE. Vision and the Aging Driver. In RG Cole, BP Rosenthal (eds), Problems in Optometry: Patient and Practice Management in Low Vision (vol 4). Philadelphia: Lippincott, 1992.

Szlyk JP, Alexander KR, Severing K. Assessment of driving performance in patients with retinitis pigmentosa. Arch Ophthalmol 1992;110:1709.

Wood JM, Troutbeck R. The effect of restriction of the binocular visual field on driving performance. Ophthalmic Physiol Optics 1992;12:291.

Barron C. Bioptic telescopic spectacles for motor vehicle driving. J Am Optom Assoc 1991;62:37.

Klein R. Age-related eye disease, visual impairment, and driving in the elderly. Hum Factors 1991;33:521.

Parisi JL, Bell RA, Yassein H. Homonymous hemianopic field defects and driving in Canada. Can J Ophthalmol 1991;26:252.

Shinar D, Schieber F. Visual requirements for safety and mobility of older drivers. Hum Factors 1991;33:507.

Spitzberg LA. A patient's experience on driving with a bioptic. J Vis Rehabil 1991;5:17.

Vogel GL. Training the bioptic telescope wearer for driving. J Am Optom Assoc 1991;62:288.

Appel SD, Brilliant RL, Reich LN. Driving with visual impairment: facts and issues. J Vis Rehabil 1990;4:19.

Bailey IL, Sheedy J. Impaired Vision and Driving. In AW Johnston, M Lawrence (eds), Low Vision Ahead II Conference Proceedings. Kooyong, Australia: Association for the Blind, 1990.

Corn AL, Lippmann O, Lewis MC. Licensed drivers with bioptic telescopic spectacles: user profiles and perceptions. RE:view 1990;21:221.

Taylor DG. Telescopic spectacles for driving: user data satisfaction, preferences and effects in vocational, educational and personal tasks: a study in Illinois. J Vis Rehabil 1990;4:29.

Goodrich GL. Driving and telescopic aids: a bibliography. J Vis Rehabil 1988;2:21.

Huss CP. Model approach—low vision driver's training and assessment. J Vis Rehabil 1988;2:31.

Lippmann O, Corn AL, Lewis AC. Bioptic telescopic spectacles and driving performance: a study in Texas. J Vis Impair Blind 1988;82:182.

Keltner JL, Johnson CA. Visual function, driving safety and the elderly. Ophthalmology 1987;94:1180.

Taylor JF. Review of vision and driving. Ophthal Physiol Optics 1987;7:200.

Fonda GF. Suggested visual standards for drivers in the United States with vision ranging from 20/175 (6/52) to 20/50 (6/15). Ann Ophthalmol 1986;18:76.

Keller S. Visually impaired drivers: is the system fair? J Wiscon Optom Assoc 1986;30:3.

Leibowitz HW, Owens DA. We drive by night. Psychol Today 1986;55(1):8.

Lovsund P, Hedin A. Effects on Driving Performance of Visual Field Defects. In AG Gale, MH Freeman, CM Haslegrave, et al. (eds), Vision in Vehicles I. Amsterdam: Elsevier, 1986;323.

Chapman BG. Techniques and variables related to driving—Part 1. J Rehabil Optom 1984;2:18.

Chapman BG. Techniques and variables related to driving—Part 2. J Rehabil Optom 1984;2:12.

Freeman PB. Visual requirements for driving. J Rehabil Optom 1984;2:6.

Huss C. A multidisciplinary approach to driving for the visually handicapped. J Rehabil Optom 1984;2:10.

Jose RT, Ousley C. The visually handicapped, driving and bioptics—some new facts. J Rehabil Optom 1984;2:2.

Padula W. The issue of driving with bioptic telescopes. J Rehabil Optom 1984;2:4.

Janke M. Accident rates of drivers with bioptic telescopes. J Safety Res 1983;14:159.

Janke M, Kazarian G. The accident record of drivers with bioptic telescopic lenses. Report #86. Sacramento, CA: State of California, Department of Public Safety—Licensing Bureau, 1983.

Jose RT. Bioptics and Driving. In Understanding Low Vision. New York: American Foundation for the Blind, 1983.

Jose RT, Carter K, Carter C. A training program for clients considering the use of bioptic telescope for driving. J Vis Impair Blind 1983;77:425.

Jose RT, Butler JH. Training a patient to drive with telescopic lenses. Am J Optom Physiol Optics 1975;152:343.

Safety Management Institute. Report on Conference on Telescopic Lens Systems and Driver Licensing. Albany, NY: Department of Motor Vehicles, 1975.

Burg A. Vision and driving: a report on research. Hum Factors 1971;58:31.

Kelleher DK, Mehr EB, Hirsch M. Motor vehicle operation by a patient with low vision. Am J Optom Physiol Optics 1971;48:773.

Burg A. Some Relationships Between Vision and Driving. In AH Keeney (ed), Proceedings of the Eleventh Annual Meeting of the American Association for Automotive Medicine. New York: Thomas, 1970.

Korb DR. Preparing the visually handicapped person for motor vehicle operation. Am J Optom Arch Am Acad Optom 1970;47:619.

MULTIPLE DISABILITIES

Allen DA, Landis RKB, Schramke CJ. The role of psychologists in the treatment of multiple sclerosis. Int J Rehabil Health 1995;1:97.

Chen D, Haney M. An early intervention model for infants who are deaf-blind. J Vis Impair Blind 1995;89:213.

Evans Luiselli T, Luiselli JK, DeCaluwe SM, Jacobs LA. Inclusive education of young children with deaf-blindness: a technical assistance model. J Vis Impair Blind 1995;89:249.

Huebner KM, Kirchner C, Prickett JG. Meeting personnel training needs: the deaf-blind self-study curriculum project. J Vis Impair Blind 1995;89:235.

Bailey GR, Downing J. Using visual accents to enhance attending symbols for students with severe multiple disabilities. RE:view 1994;26:101.

Odess B, Margaliot S. Creating appropriate toys for children with multiple handicaps. RE:view 1994;26:35.

Bailey BR, Head DN. Providing O&M services to children and youth with severe multiple disabilities. RE:view 1993;25:57.

Bolduc M, Gresset J, Sanschagrin S, Thibodeau J. A model for the efficient interdisciplinary assessment of young visually impaired children. J Vis Impair Blind 1993;87:410.

Bowden J, Thorburn J. Including a student with multiple disabilities and visual impairment in her neighborhood school. J Vis Impair Blind 1993;87:268.

Haegerstrom-Portnoy G. New procedures for evaluating vision functions of special populations. Optom Vis Sci 1993;70:306.

Kelley P, Davidson R, Sanspree MJ. Vision and orientation and mobility consultation for children with severe multiple disabilities. J Vis Impair Blind 1993;87:397.

Lolli D. Orientation and mobility for low vision and multihandicapped children. In Proceedings of the 6th International Mobility Conference (vol II). Madrid: Spanish National Organization of the Blind, 1993;315.

Nielsen L. Early learning, step by step in children with vision impairment and multiple disabilities. Copenhagen, Denmark: Sikon, 1993.

Chen D, Smith J. Developing orientation and mobility skills in students who are multihandicapped and visually impaired. RE:view 1992;24:133.

Geruschat DR. Using the acuity card procedure to assess visual acuity in children with severe and multiple impairments. J Vis Impair Blind 1992;86:25.

Hinrichs CA. Vision rehabilitation for the multiply challenged child. J Optom Vis Dev 1992;23:9.

Jaworski CN. Preferential looking visual acuity assessment in handicapped children. J Vis Rehabil, 1992;6:1.

Michael MG, Paul PV. Early intervention for infants with deafblindness. Except Children 1991;57:200.

Morse MT. Augmenting assessment procedures for children with severe multiple handicaps and sensory impairments. J Vis Impair Blind 1992;86:73.

Ogden NA, Raymond JE, Seland TP. Visual accommodation and sustained visual resolution in multiple sclerosis. Invest Ophthalmol Vis Sci 1992;33:2744.

Rogow SM. Visual perceptual problems of visually impaired children with developmental disabilities. RE:view 1992;24:57.

van Diemen HAM, van Dongen MMMM, Dammers JWHH, et al. Increased visual impairment after exercise (Uhthoff's phenomenon) in multiple sclerosis: therapeutic possibilities. Eur Neurol 1992;32:231.

Zambone AM, Huebner KM. Services for children and youths who are deaf-blind: an overview. J Vis Impair Blind 1992;86:287.

Aitken S, Buultjens M. Visual assessments of children with multiple impairments: a survey of ophthalmologists. J Vis Impair Blind 1991;85:170.

Hall A, Orel-Bixler D, Haegerstrom-Portnoy G. Special visual assessment techniques for multiply handicapped persons. J Vis Impair Blind 1991;85:23.

Jackson AJ, Morrison E, O'Donoghue E, et al. The provision of ophthalmic services for a rehabilitation day centre population with multiple physical handicaps. Ophthalmic Physiol Optics 1991;11:314.

Joffee E, Rikhye CH. Orientation and mobility for students with severe visual and multiple impairments: a new perspective. J Vis Impair Blind 1991;85:211.

Morse M. Visual gaze behaviors: considerations in working with visually impaired multiply handicapped children. RE:view 1991;23:5.

Downing J, Bailey B. Developing vision use within functional daily activities for students with visual and multiple disabilities. RE:view 1990;21:209.

Erin J, Daugherty W, Dignax K, et al. Teachers of visually handicapped students with multiple disabilities: perceptions of adequacy. J Vis Impair Blind 1990;84:16.

Hyvarinen L, Gimble L, Sorri M. Assessment of vision and hearing of deaf-blind persons. Burwood, Australia: Royal Victorian Institute for the Blind, 1990.

Maino JH. Mental retardation syndromes with associated ocular defects. J Am Optom Assoc 1990;9:707.

Morse MT. Cortical visual impairment in young children with multiple disabilities. J Vis Impair Blind 1990;84:200.

Osborn R. The Value of Assessing and Understanding Functional Aspects of Hearing Loss in Older Visually Impaired People. In AW Johnston, M Lawrence (eds), Low Vision Ahead II Conference Proceedings. Kooyong, Australia: Association for the Blind, 1990.

Placha J. Providing services for multiply impaired persons. J Vis Impair Blind 1990;84:88.

Stiefel DH. The Madness of Usher's. Corpus Christi, TX: Business of Living Publications, 1990.

Erin J (ed). Dimensions: Selected Papers from The Journal of Visual Impairment and Blindness on Visually Impaired Persons with Multiple Disabilities. New York: American Foundation for the Blind, 1989.

Hammer E. Research Issues in Educating Visually Handicapped Persons with Multiple Impairments. In MC Wang, MC Reynolds, HJ Walberg (eds), Handbook of Special Education: Research and Practice (vol 3). New York: Pergamon, 1990.

Johnson SK, Corn AL. The past, present, and future of education for gifted children with sensory and/or physical disabilities. RE:view 1989;12:13.

Orel-Bixler D, Haegerstrom-Portnoy G, Hall A. Visual assessment of the multiply handicapped patient. Optom Vis Sci 1989;66:530.

Ronis MG. Optometric care for the handicapped. Optom Vis Sci 1989;66:12.

Clarke K. Barriers or enablers? Mobility devices for visually impaired multihandicapped infants and preschoolers. Educ Vis Handicapped 1988;20:115.

Duncan E, Prickett HT, Finkelstein D, et al. Usher's Syndrome: What It Is, How to Cope, and How to Help. Springfield, IL: Thomas, 1988.

Erhardt RP, Beatty PA, Hertsgaard DM. A developmental visual assessment for children with multiple handicaps. Top Early Childhood Educ 1988;7:84.

Birch E, Hale L, Stager D, et al. Operant acuity of toddlers and developmentally delayed children with low vision. J Pediatr Ophthalmol Strabismus 1987;24:64.

Buultjens M, Aitken S. Assessment of vision in multiply impaired children—a consideration of evidence. Br J Special Educ 1987;141:12.

Gee K, Harrell K, Rosenberg R. Teaching Orientation and Mobility Skills Within and Across Natural Opportunities in Travel. In L Goetz, D Guess, K Stemel-Campbell (eds), Innovative Program Design for Individuals with Dual Sensory Impairments. Baltimore: Brookes, 1987.

Hyvarinen L. Assessment of Vision of Deaf-Blind Persons. In GC Woo (ed), Low Vision: Principles and Applications. New York: Springer, 1987.

Sisson LA, Van Hasselt VB, Hersen M. Psychological approaches with deaf-blind persons: strategies and issues in research and treatment. Clin Psychol Rev 1987;7:303.

Zahn J. Usher's syndrome: psychological and electrodiagnostic data on three families. J Vis Rehabil 1987;1:15.

Bell J. An approach to the stimulation of vision in the pro-foundly handicapped visually handicapped child. Br J Vis Impair 1986;4:46.

Ellis D. Sensory impairments in mentally handicapped people. London: Croom Helm, 1986.

Scheiman M. Optometric findings in children with cerebral palsy. Am J Optom Physiol Optics 1984;61:321.

Cote KS, Smith A. Assessment of the Multiply Handicapped. In RT Jose (ed), Understanding Low Vision. New York: American Foundation for the Blind, 1983.

Piccolo M, Jose RT. Contact lenses for the multiply impaired. J Rehabil Optom 1983;1:7.

Smith AJ, Cote KS. Look at Me: A Resource Manual for the Development of Residual Vision in Multiply Impaired Children. Philadelphia: College of Optometry Press, 1982.

Geruschat DR. Orientation and mobility for the low functioning deaf-blind child. J Vis Impair Blind 1980;74:29.

Harley RK, Merbler JB. Development of an orientation and mobility program for multiply impaired low vision children. J Vis Impair Blind 1980;74:9.

Jose RT, Smith AJ, Shane KG. Evaluating and stimulating vision in the multiply impaired. J Vis Impair Blind 1980;74:2.

Ficociello C. Techniques of Teaching Deaf-Blind Children. Dallas, TX: South Central Regional Center for Services to Deaf-Blind Children, 1976.

PRISM

Gottlieb DD, Freeman P, Williams M. Clinical research and statistical analysis of a visual field awareness system. J Am Optom Assoc 1992;63:581.

Lapidow FM. An alternate use of prisms for field enhancement. J Vis Rehabil 1992;6:4.

Perlin RR, Dziadul J. Fresnel prisms for field enhancement of patients with constricted or hemianopic visual fields. J Am Optom Assoc 1991;621:58.

Weiss NJ. An unusual application of prisms for field enhancement. J Am Optom Assoc 1990;61:291.

Rosenberg R, Gaye E, Fischer M, Budick D. Role of prism relocation in improving visual performance of patients with macular dysfunction. Optom Vis Sci 1989;66:747.

Spitzberg L, Jose RT, Kuether C. A new ergonomically designed prism stand magnifier. J Vis Rehabil 1989;3:47.

Weiss NJ. An unusual application of cemented prisms. J Am Optom Assoc 1989;60:291.

Brilliant RL. The Amorphic Fresnel Prism Trioptical System. In G Woo (ed), Low Vision: Principles and Applications. New York: Springer, 1987.

Edmonds S, Edmonds SE. Prismatic scanning vs. standard microscope techniques. J Vis Rehabil 1987;1:149.

Cohen J, Waiss B. Vertical yoked prisms—a low vision mobility aid. J Rehabil Optom 1984;Fall:5.

Bailey IL. Can prisms control eccentric viewing. Optom Monthly 1983;74:360.

White JM, Jose RT, Bedell HE. Eccentric viewing with prism—speculations. J Rehabil Optom 1983;Spring:14.

Woo GC, Mandelman T. Fresnel prism therapy for right hemianopia. Am J Optom Physiol Optics 1983;60:739.

Ferraro J, Jose RT, McClain L. Fresnel prisms as a treatment option for retinitis pigmentosa. Tex Optom 1982;38:13.

Romayananda N, Wong SW, Elzeneiny IH, Chan GH. Prismatic scanning method for improving visual acuity in patients with low vision. Ophthalmology 1982;89:937.

Hoffman L, Soden R. Inferior altitudinal losses and prismatic correction. J Am Optom Assoc 1981;52:818.

Bailey IL. Prismatic treatment for field defects. Optom Monthly 1978;69:73.

Gadbaw P, Finn W, Dolan M, De l'Aune W. Parameters of success in the use of Fresnel prisms. Opt J Rev Optom 1976;113:41.

Jose RT, Smith AJ. Increasing peripheral field awareness with Fresnel prisms. Opt J Rev Optom 1976;113:33.

Finn WA, Gadbaw PO, Kevorkian CA, De l'Aune WR. Increased field accessibility through prismatically displaced images. New Outlook for the Blind 1975;69:465.

Freidman G. Prisms to enlarge the visual field. Low Vision Clinical Society (special supplement). Near Point 1975;1(2):3.

Hoeft W. Mirrors, Prisms, Eccentric Field Defects. In E Faye (ed), Low Vision. Springfield, IL: Thomas, 1975.

Weiss NJ. An application of cemented prisms with severe field loss. Am J Optom Physiol Optics 1972;49:261.

Gostin S. Ambulation-prism-spectacles. Am Acad Ophthalmol Otolaryngol Trans 1971;75:644.

Young CA. Homonymous hemianopsia during pregnancy aided by reflecting prisms. Arch Ophthalmol 1929;2:560.

Baunschwig P. Hemianopsia aided by prisms. Ophthalmol Yearbook 1922;395.

PSYCHOSOCIAL ASSESSMENT

Davis C, Lovie-Kitchin J, Thompson B. Psychosocial adjustment to age-related macular degeneration. J Vis Impair Blind 1995;89:16.

Jackson R, Lawson G. Family environment and psychological distress in persons who are visually impaired. J Vis Impair Blind 1995;89:157.

Miner ID. Psychosocial implications of Usher syndrome, Type I, throughout the life cycle. J Vis Impair Blind 1995;89:287.

Brenner MH, Curbow B, Javitt JC. Vision change and quality of life in the elderly: response to cataract surgery and treatment of other chronic ocular conditions. Arch Ophthalmol 1993;111:680.

Dodds A. Rehabilitating Blind and Visually Impaired People: A Psychological Approach. London: Chapman & Hall, 1993.

Dodds AG, Bailey P, Pearson A, Yates L. Multi-Dimensional Aspects of Emotional Adjustment to Acquired Visual Loss: A Cognitive Alternative to the Loss Model. In Proceedings of the 6th International Mobility Conference (vol II). Madrid: Spanish National Organization of the Blind, 1993;82.

Kelley SDM, Tedder NE. Serving persons with both psychiatric and vision disabilities in psychosocial rehabilitation. Psychosocial Rehabil J 1993;16:101.

Lane SD, Mikhail BI, Reizian A, et al. Sociocultural aspects of blindness in an Egyptian Delta hamlet: visual impairment vs. visual disability. Med Anthropol 1993;15:245.

Wulsin LR, Jacobson AM, Rand LI. Psychosocial adjustments to advanced proliferative diabetic retinopathy. Diabetes Care 1993;16:1061.

Agrawal R. Psychosocial factors in mainstreaming visually impaired adults. J Vis Impair Blind 1992;86:119.

Beggs WDA. Coping, adjustment, and mobility-related feelings of newly visually impaired young adults. J Vis Impair Blind 1992;86:136.

Melzack R. Phantom limbs. Sci Am 1992;266:120.

Needham WE, Taylor RE. Benign visual hallucinations, or "phantom vision" in visually impaired and blind persons. J Vis Impair Blind 1992;86:245.

Beatty LA. The effects of visual impairment on adolescents' self-concept. J Vis Impair Blind 1991;85:129.

Dodds AG. Psychological assessment and the rehabilitation process. The New Beacon 1991;25:101.

Dodds AG, Bailey P, Pearson A, Yates L. Psychological factors in acquired visual impairment: the development of a scale of adjustment. J Vis Impair Blind 1991;85:306.

Wiemer SA, Kratochwill TR. Fears of visually impaired children. J Vis Impair Blind 1991;85:118.

Biaggio MK, Bittner E. Psychology and optometry: interaction and collaboration. Am Psychol 1990;45:1313.

Drummond MF (ed). Measuring the Quality of Life of People with Visual Impairment: Proceedings of a Workshop (Publication No. 90-3078). Bethesda, MD: National Institutes of Health, 1990.

Ringering L, Amaral P. Vision Loss in the Elderly: Psychological Repercussions and Interventions. In AW Johnston, M Lawrence (eds), Low Vision Ahead II Conference Proceedings. Kooyong, Australia: Association for the Blind, 1990.

Agrawal R, Piplani R. Alienation among the visually impaired: some important predictors. J Psychol 1989;123:517.

Allen MN. The meaning of visual impairment to visually impaired adults. J Adv Nurs 1989;14:640.

Gold K, Rabins PV. Isolated visual hallucinations and the Charles Bonnet syndrome. Comp Psychiatry 1989;30:90.

Klebaner RP. Bridge counseling: from medical diagnosis to rehabilitation readiness. J Vis Rehabil 1989;3:37.

Lankhorst GJ. Quality of life: an exploratory study. Int J Rehabil Res 1989;12:201.

Obiakor FE, Stile SW. Enhancing self-concept in students with visual handicaps. J Vis Impair Blind 1989;83:255.

Warren D. Implications of Visual Impairments for Child Development. In MC Wang, MC Reynolds, HJ Walberg (eds), Handbook of Special Education: Research and Practice, Vol 3: Low Incidence. New York: Pergamon, 1989.

Wyatt WJ, Swick DR, Huss CP. The psychologist's role in low vision driver evaluation. J Vis Rehabil 1989;3:39.

Crespi TD. Coping in the dark: counseling adults with visual impairments. Counselor Educ Supervision 1988;28:146.

Tobin MJ, Hill EW. Visually impaired teenagers: ambitions, attitudes, and interests. J Vis Impair Blind 1988;82:414.

Carnes GD. Psychological assessment by the visually disabled psychologist. Clin Psychol 1987;40:40.

Jan JE, Groenveld JE, Sykanda AM, Hoyt CS. Behavioral characteristics of children with permanent cortical visual impairment. Dev Med Child Neurol 1987;29:571.

Olbrich HM, Engelmeier MP, Pauleikhoff D, Waubke T. Visual hallucinations in ophthalmology. Graefes Arch Clin Exp Ophthalmol 1987;225:217.

Price JR, Mount GR, Coles EA. Evaluating the visually impaired: neuropsychological techniques. J Vis Impair Blind 1987;81:28.

Rosenbaum F, Harati Y, Rolak L. Visual hallucinations in sane people: the Charles Bonnet syndrome. J Am Geriatr Soc 1987;35:66.

Santangelo M, Overbury O, Lang R. Life Satisfaction of Low Vision Patients and Other Disability Groups: A Preliminary Study. In GC Woo (ed), Low Vision: Principles and Applications. New York: Springer, 1987.

Taylor DG. Models of psychosocial adjustment to physical and sensory disabilities. J Vis Rehabil 1987;1:27.

VanderKolk CJ. Psychosocial Assessment of Visually Impaired Persons. In B Heller, L Flohr, LS Zegans (eds), Psychosocial Interventions with Sensorially Disabled Persons. San Francisco: Grune & Stratton, 1987.

Ammerman R, Van Hasselt V, Hersen M. Psychological adjustment of visually handicapped children and youth. Clin Psychol Rev 1986;6:67.

Greig DE, West ML, Overbury O. Successful use of low vision aids: visual and psychological factors. J Vis Impair Blind 1986;80:985.

Hall A, Scholl GT, Swallow RM. Psychoeducational Assessment. In GT Scholl (ed), Foundations of Education for Blind and Visually Handicapped Children and Youth: Theory and Practice. New York: American Foundation for the Blind, 1986.

Nemshick LA, Vernon M, Ludman F. The impact of retinitis pigmentosa on young adults: psychological, educational, vocational and social considerations. J Vis Impair Blind 1986;80:859.

Taylor RE, Mancil GL, Kramer SH. Visual hallucinations: meaning and management. J Am Optom Assoc 1986;57:889.

Agrawal R, Kaur J. Anxiety and adjustment levels among the visually and hearing impaired and their relationship to locus of control, cognitive social, and biographical variables. J Psychol 1985;119:265.

Shindell S. A Summary of Current Psychosocial Research in Blindness and Visual Impairment. In GL Goodrich (ed), Yearbook of the Association for Education of the Blind and Visually Impaired. Washington, DC: Association for Education of the Blind and Visually Impaired, 1985.

Morse JL. Psychosocial Aspects of Low Vision. In RT Jose (ed), Understanding Low Vision. New York: American Foundation for the Blind, 1983.

Negrin S. Psychosocial Aspects of Aging and Visual Impairment. In RT Jose (ed), Understanding Low Vision. New York: American Foundation for the Blind, 1983.

Berrios GE, Brook P. The Charles Bonnet syndrome and the problem of visual perceptual disorders in the elderly. Age Ageing 1982;11:17.

Keane JR. Neuro-ophthalmic signs and symptoms of hysteria. Neurology 1982;32:757.

Lowenfeld B. Psychological Problems of Children with Severely Impaired Vision. In W Cruickshank (ed), Psychology of Exceptional Children and Youth. Englewood Cliffs, NJ: Prentice-Hall, 1980.

Morse J. Psycho-Social Aspects of Low Vision: Considerations and Interventions. In M Beliveau, A Smith (eds), The Interdisciplinary Approach to Low Vision Rehabilitation. Washington, DC: Rehabilitation Services Administration, 1980.

Mehr HM. Psychological aspects of low vision care. J Nat Assoc Educ Partially Sighted 1977;Summer:4.

Bauman MK. Psychological and Educational Assessment. In B Lowenfeld (ed), The Visually Handicapped Child in School. London: Constable, 1974.

Mehr EB. Psychological Factors in Low Vision Care. In JD Newman (ed), A Guide to the Care of Low Vision Patients. St. Louis: American Optometric Association, 1974.

Mehr EB, Mehr HM. Psychological factors in working with the partially sighted. Optician 1972;164:424.

Mehr EB, Mehr HM, Ault C. Psychological aspects of low vision rehabilitation. Am J Optom Arch Am Acad Optom 1970;47:605.

Valvo A. Behavior patterns and visual rehabilitation after early and long-lasting blindness. Am J Ophthalmol 1968;65:19.

Cholden LS. A Psychiatrist Works with Blindness. New York: American Foundation for the Blind, 1958.

TRAINING

Waiss B, Cohen JM. Visual Impairment and Visual Efficiency Training. In RG Cole, BP Rosenthal (eds), Remediation and Management of Low Vision. St. Louis: Mosby–Year Book, 1996;59.

Donohue B, Acierno R, Van Hasselt VB, Hersen M. Social skills training in a depressed, visually impaired older adult. J Behav Ther Exp Psychiatry 1995;26:65.

Jose R. Clinical wisdoms. Home training for eccentric viewing. J Vis Rehabil 1995;9:4

Kozel B. Diabetes and orientation and mobility training: an added challenge. J Vis Impair Blind 1995;89:337.

Park WL, Unatin J, Park JM. A profile of the demographics, training and driving history of telescopic drivers in the state of Michigan. J Am Optom Assoc 1995;66:274.

Stoll S, Sarma S, Hoeft WW. Low vision aids training in the home. J Am Optom Assoc 1995;66:32.

White KD, Saravanabhavan RC. Intensive training program to enhance life skills among people who are visually impaired. J Vis Impair Blind 1995;89:170.

Backman O. Reading Skills, Reading Training and Technology for the Visually Handicapped—Prospects of the 1990s. In AC Kooijman, PL Looijestijn, JA Welling, GJ van der Wildt (eds), Low Vision: Research and New Developments in Rehabilitation. Amsterdam: International Optical Society Press, 1994;251.

Bozic N. How Should Computers be Used in the Visual Training of Young Visually Impaired Children? In AC Kooijman, PL Looijestijn, JA Welling, GJ van der Wildt (eds), Low Vision: Research and New Developments in Rehabilitation. Amsterdam: International Optical Society Press, 1994;334.

Cheung SYM. O&M Training for the Multi-Handicapped in Hong Kong. In G Clarke, T Heyes (eds), Visions in Mobility: Proceedings of the International Mobility Conference 7. Kew, Australia: Royal Guide Dogs Associations of Australia, 1994;107.

Clarke G. Functional Assessment, Evaluation and Training of Low Vision Elderly Clients in Residential Accommodation. In G Clarke, T Heyes (eds), Visions in Mobility: Proceedings of the International Mobility Conference 7. Kew, Australia: Royal Guide Dogs Associations of Australia, 1994;162.

Dodds AG. Low Vision Assessment and Training: The Use of Computer Generated Graphics. In G Clarke, T Heyes (eds), Visions in Mobility: Proceedings of the International Mobility Conference 7. Kew, Australia: Royal Guide Dogs Associations of Australia, 1994;40.

Fitzmaurice K, Kinnear JF, Chen YA. ECCVUE: A Computer Generated Method of Training Eccentric Viewing. In AC Kooijman, PL Looijestijn, JA Welling, GJ van der Wildt (eds), Low Vision: Research and New Developments in Rehabilitation. Amsterdam: International Optical Society Press, 1994;283.

Ighe S. Reading Training—Four Cases. In AC Kooijman, PL Looijestijn, JA Welling, GJ van der Wildt (eds), Low Vision: Research and New Developments in Rehabilitation. Amsterdam: International Optical Society Press, 1994;225.

Joosten-Room H, Bouw W, Roorda N. Lists of Steps for A.D.L. Training. In AC Kooijman, PL Looijestijn, JA Welling, GJ van der Wildt (eds), Low Vision: Research and New Developments in Rehabilitation. Amsterdam: International Optical Society Press, 1994;452.

Keeffe J, Lawrence M, Lovie-Kitchin J, et al. Low Vision Assessment and Training Materials for Use in Developing Countries. In AC Kooijman, PL Looijestijn, JA Welling, GJ van der Wildt (eds), Low Vision: Research and New Developments in Rehabilitation. Amsterdam: International Optical Society Press, 1994;47.

Levitt JG, Ighe S. Optometric Involvement in Low Vision Training. In AC Kooijman, PL Looijestijn, JA Welling, GJ van der Wildt (eds), Low Vision: Research and New Developments in Rehabilitation. Amsterdam: International Optical Society Press, 1994;584.

Martinsen H, Storliliokken M, Elmerskog B, Tellevik JM. Functional Mobility Training of Multiple Disabled Blind Children and Adults. In G Clarke, T Heyes (eds), Visions in Mobility: Proceedings of the International Mobility Conference 7. Kew, Australia: Royal Guide Dogs Associations of Australia, 1994;266.

Nilsson SEG, Nilsson UL. Educational Training in the Use of Aids and Residual Vision is Essential in Rehabilitation of Patients with Severe Age-Related Macular Degeneration. I. Principles and Methods. In AC Kooijman, PL Looijestijn, JA Welling, GJ van der Wildt (eds), Low Vision: Research and New Developments in Rehabilitation. Amsterdam: International Optical Society Press, 1994;147.

Sands L. Evaluation of a Training Program Designed to Improve Mobility Skills for People with Homonymous Hemianopia. In G Clarke, T Heyes (eds), Visions in Mobility: Proceedings of the International Mobility Conference 7. Kew, Australia: Royal Guide Dogs Associations of Australia, 1994;294.

Vallender M. Developing Visual Training Programs on an IBM PC Compatible Microcomputer. In AC Kooijman, PL Looijestijn, JA Welling, GJ van der Wildt (eds), Low Vision: Research and New Developments in Rehabilitation. Amsterdam: International Optical Society Press, 1994;331.

Blakely KS, Lang MA (eds). AIDS, Blindness, and Low Vision: A Training Manual for Health Organizations. New York: The Lighthouse Inc, 1993.

Tavernier GGF. The improvement of vision by vision stimulation and training: a review of the literature. J Vis Impair Blind 1993;87:143.

Fraser KE. Training the Low Vision Patient. In RG Cole, BP Rosenthal (eds), Problems in Optometry: Patient and Practice Management in Low Vision (vol 4). Philadelphia: Lippincott, 1992.

Watson GR, Wright V, De l'Aune W. The efficacy of comprehension training and reading practice for print readers with macular loss. J Vis Impair Blind 1992;86:37.

Zimmerman GJ. Orientation and mobility training: enhancing the employment prospects for persons with blindness and visual impairments. J Voc Rehabil 1992;2:66.

Vogel GL. Training the bioptic telescope wearer for driving. J Am Optom Assoc 1991;62:288.

Walls MK, Molenda MM. Training procedures for more cosmetically appealing miniaturized telescopes. J Vis Rehabil 1991;5:11.

Buser F. Practical Experiences in Low Vision Training. In AW Johnston, M Lawrence (eds), Low Vision Ahead II Conference Proceedings. Kooyong, Australia: Association for the Blind, 1990.

Culham L, Silver J, Bird A. Assessment of Low Vision Training in Age-Related Macular Disease. In AW Johnston, M Lawrence (eds), Low Vision Ahead II Conference Proceedings. Kooyong, Australia: Association for the Blind, 1990.

Goodrich GL. Perceptual Implications in Vision Rehabilitation Training. In AW Johnston, M Lawrence (eds), Low Vision Ahead II Conference Proceedings. Kooyong, Australia: Association for the Blind, 1990.

Mettler R. An integrated, problem-solving approach to low vision training. J Vis Impair Blind 1990;84:171.

Nilsson UL. Visual rehabilitation with and without educational training in the use of optical aids and residual vision. Clin Vis Sci 1990;6:3.

Trudeau M, Overbury O, Conrod B. Perceptual training and figure-ground performance in low vision. J Vis Impair Blind 1990;84:204.

Watson GR, De l'Aune WR. Computerized Eccentric Viewing Assistant for Training Eccentric Viewing and Reading. In AW Johnston, M Lawrence (eds), Low Vision Ahead II Conference Proceedings. Kooyong, Australia: Association for the Blind, 1990.

Aston SJ. Short-term training vision and aging project. Educ Gerontol 1989;15:415.

Dodds AG, Davis DP. Assessment and training of low vision clients for mobility. J Vis Impair Blind 1989;83:439.

Hall A, Bailey IL. A model for training vision function. J Vis Impair Blind 1989;83:390.

Watson G, De l'Aune W, Ehrnst W, Blair J. Development of the family training program curriculum in low vision. J Rehabil Res Dev 1989;26:372.

Beggs WDA. Different Approaches to Training the Low-Vision Client. In N Neustadt-Noy, S Merin, Y Schiff (eds), Orientation & Mobility of the Visually Impaired. Jerusalem: Heiliger Publishing, 1988.

Dodds A. Mobility Training for Visually Handicapped People: A Person-Centered Approach. London: Croom Helm, 1988.

Dodds AG, Davies D. Low Vision: Functional Assessment and Training. In N Neustadt-Noy, S Merin, Y Schiff (eds), Orientation and Mobility of the Visually Impaired. Jerusalem: Heiliger Publishing, 1988.

Huss CP. Model approach—low vision driver's training and assessment. J Vis Rehabil 1988;2:31.

O'Donnell BA. Stress and mobility training process: a literature review. J Vis Impair Blind 1988;82:143.

Faubert J, Overbury O, Goodrich GL. A Hierarchy of Perceptual Training in Low Vision. In GC Woo (ed), Low Vision: Principles and Applications. New York: Springer, 1987.

Goodrich GL, Mehr EB. Eccentric viewing training and low vision aids: current practice and implications of peripheral retinal research. Am J Optom Physiol Optics 1986;63:119.

Peli E. Control of eye movement with peripheral vision: implications for training of eccentric viewing. Am J Optom Physiol Optics 1986;63:113.

Goodrich GL, Overbury O, Mehr EB, Harsh M. A low vision training manual—the VETBook. Invest Ophthalmol Vis Sci (Suppl) 1985;26:219.

Frere S. Comprehensive Programs for the Visually Handicapped: Low Vision Training Materials from the American Printing House for the Blind. Louisville, KY: American Printing House for the Blind, 1984.

Maplesden C. A subjective approach to eccentric viewing training. J Vis Impair Blind 1984;78:5.

Berg RV, Jose RT, Carter K. Distance Training Techniques. In RT Jose (ed), Understanding Low Vision. New York: American Foundation for the Blind, 1983.

Ferraro J, Jose RT. Training Programs for Individuals with Restricted Fields. In RT Jose (ed), Understanding Low Vision. New York: American Foundation for the Blind, 1983.

Ferraro S, Ferraro J. Establishing a Training-Instructional Program. In RT Jose (ed), Understanding Low Vision. New York: American Foundation for the Blind, 1983.

Jose RT, Browning R. Training with the expanded field bioptic telescope. J Rehabil Optom 1983;1:5.

Jose RT, Carter K, Carter C. A training program for clients considering the use of bioptic telescope for driving. J Vis Impair Blind 1983;77:425.

Watson G, Berg RV. Near Training Techniques. In RT Jose (ed), Understanding Low Vision. New York: American Foundation for the Blind, 1983.

Geruschat D. Training with Hand-Held Distance Optical Aids. In M Beliveau, A Smith (eds), The Interdisciplinary Approach to Low Vision Rehabilitation. Washington, DC: Rehabilitation Services Administration, 1980.

Hoeft W. Bioptic telescopes: training and adaptation. Optom Monthly 1980;9:71.

Inde K. Low Vision Training as an Educational Model in Sweden. Low Vision Rehabilitation II. Uppsala, Sweden: Department of Education, University of Uppsala, 1980.

Lederer J, Wulff J. Vision Training. In Low Vision Ahead, Proceedings of the First Australian Pacific Conference on Low Vision. Melbourne, Australia: Association for the Blind, 1980.

Quillman RD. Low Vision Training Manual. Kalamazoo, MI: Western Michigan University, 1980.

Inde K. Low vision training in Sweden. J Vis Impair Blind 1978;72:307.

Newman JD, Pogoda A. An overview of visual rehabilitation and training of the low vision patient. J Am Optom Assoc 1978;49:423.

Overbury O, Bross M. Visual training for the severely impaired: implications of research findings to applied situations. Low Vis Abs 1978;4:7.

Goodrich GL, Mehr EB, Quillman RD, et al. Training and practice effects in performance with low vision aids: a preliminary study. Am J Optom Physiol Optics 1977;54:312.

Goodrich GL, Quillman RD. Training eccentric viewing. J Vis Impair Blind 1977;71:377.

Holcomb JG, Goodrich GL. Eccentric viewing training. J Am Optom Assoc 1976;47:1438.

Watson G, Jose RT. A training sequence for low vision patients. J Am Optom Assoc 1976;47:1407.

Jose RT, Butler J. Driver's training for partially sighted persons: an interdisciplinary approach. New Outlook Blind 1975;69:305.

Jose RT, Butler JH. Training a patient to drive with telescopic lenses. Am J Optom Physiol Optics 1975;52:343.

Appendix E: Organizations Involved with Low Vision

Achromatopsia Network
P.O. Box 214
Berkeley, CA 94701-0214
(510) 540-4700

American Council of the Blind
1010 Vermont Avenue NW, Suite 100
Washington, DC 20005
(202) 393-3666

American Diabetes Association
1660 Duke Street
Alexandria, VA 22314
(703) 549-1500

American Foundation for the Blind
15 West 16th Street
New York, NY 10011
(800) 232-5463
This organization can provide telephone numbers of regional offices.

American Printing House for the Blind
P.O. Box 6085
1839 Frankfort Avenue
Louisville, KY 40206
(502) 895-2485

Association for the Education and Rehabilitation
  of the Blind and Visually Impaired
206 North Washington Street, Suite 320
Alexandria, VA 22314
(703) 548-1884

Association for Macular Disease
210 East 64th Street
New York, NY 10021
(212) 605-3719

Association of Radio Reading Services
P.O. Box 847
Lawrence, KS 66044
(913) 864-4600

Council of Citizens with Low Vision, International
1357 East David Road
Kettering, OH 45429-5703
(513) 294-0533

Helen Keller National Center for Deaf-Blind Youths and Adults
111 Middle Neck Road
Sands Point, NY 11050
(516) 944-0900 (voice and TDD)

Library of Congress National Library Services
   for the Blind and Physically Handicapped
1291 Taylor Street NW
Washington, DC 20542
(202) 287-5100; (800) 424-9100

Macular Degeneration International
2968 West Ina Road #106
Tucson, AZ 85741
(520) 797-2525

National Association for the Visually Handicapped
22 West 21st Street
New York, NY 10010
(212) 889-3141

National Organization for Albinism and Hypopigmentation
Nevil Institute for Rehabilitation
919 Walnut Street, Room 400
Philadelphia, PA 19107
(215) 627-3501

National Society to Prevent Blindness
500 East Remmington Road
Schaumburg, IL 60173
(312) 843-2020

Appendix F: Manufacturers and Distributors of Low Vision Devices

Manufacturer	Product
Ai Squared P.O. Box 669 Manchester Center, VT 05255 (802) 362-3612	Computer software
Art Optical Contact Lens, Inc. 3175 Three Mile Road NW Grand Rapids, MI 49501 (800) 253-9364	Contact lenses
Beecher Research Company 906 Morse Avenue Schaumburg, IL 60193 (708) 893-0187	Binoculars
Bernell Corporation 750 Lincolnway East, Box 4637 South Bend, IN 46634 (800) 348-2225	Optical low vision devices Diagnostic equipment
C.O.I.L. Combined Optical Industries, Ltd. 1850 Howard Street Elk Grove Village, IL 60007 (800) 933-COIL	Full line of optical and nonoptical devices
Corning Medical Optics P.O. Box 1511 Elmira, NY 14902-1511 (800) 742-5273	Absorptive lenses

Designs for Vision, Inc.
760 Koehler Avenue
Ronkonkoma, NY 11779
(800) 345-4009

Microscopes, bioptics, surgical telescopes, charts, full line of optical devices
Low vision instructional services

Donegan Optical
15549 West 108th Street
Lenexa, KS 66215
(913) 492-2500

Magnifiers

Edroy Products Company, Inc.
245 North Midland Ave
Nyack, NY 10096
(800) 033-8803

Magnifiers

Edwards Optical Corporation
P.O. Box 3299
Virginia Beach, VA 23454
(800) 452-5988

Bioptics

Enhanced Vision Systems
2915 Redhill Avenue, Suite B201
Costa Mesa, CA 92626
(800) 440-9476

V-max

Eschenbach Optik of America, Inc.
904 Ethan Allen Highway
Ridgefield, CT 06877
(202) 438-7471

Full line of optical and nonoptical devices
Low vision instructional services

F/V Microscopes
1500 Broadhead Road
Aliquippa, PA 15001
(412) 375-7030

Volk lenses
Low vision instructional services

Goodkin and Associates
4918 Shamrock Court
Mableton, GA 30059
(800) 759-6275

Full line of optical and nonoptical devices

HumanWare
6404 Dry Bend Cove
Austin, TX 78731
(512) 452-5180

Closed-circuit televisions

Innoventions, Inc. 5921 South Middlefield Road, #102 Littleton, CO 80123-2877 (800) 854-6554	Magni-Cam
In-Wave Optics, Inc. 29 West Milwaukee Sreet Janesville, WI 53545 (800) 957-8400	Prism system
Keeler Optical Products, Inc. 1456 Parkway Avenue Broomall, PA 19008 (800) 523-5620	Full line of spectacle-mounted optical devices
Luzerne Optical 180 North Wilkes-Barre Boulevard Wilkes-Barre, PA 18703 (800) 223-9637 (national) (800) 432-8096 (in PA)	Spectacle microscopes
M-Tech Optics Corporation 4515 North Woodward Avenue Royal Oak, MI 48073 (313) 266-2181	Panavex telescopes
Mattingly International 938 K Andreason Drive Escondido, CA 92029 (800) 826-4200	Full line of optical and nonoptical devices Low vision instructional services
Mentor, O&O 3000 Longwater Drive Norwell, MA 02061 (800) 992 7557	Scrolling closed-circuit televisions
Microsystems Software, Inc. 600 Worcester Road Framingham, MA 01702 (800) 828-2600	Software
Mons International 800 Peachtree Street NE, Suite 200 Atlanta, GA 30308 (404) 344-8805	Full line of optical and nonoptical devices

Nikon Optics 1300 Walt Whitman Road Melville, NY 11747 (800) 645-6678	Spectacle microscopes and telescopic devices
NOIR Medical Technologies P.O. Box 159 South Lyon, MI 48178 (800) 521-9746 (USA) (800) 227-3396 (Canada)	Absorptive wrap for lenses
Ocutech, Inc. 143 West Franklin Street, Suite 203 Chapel Hill, NC 27516 (800) 326-6460	Bioptic telescopes, auto-focus telescopes, minifiers
Okaya Electronic America, Inc. 503 Wall Street Valparaiso, IN 46383 (800) 325-4488	Closed-circuit televisions
Optelec, Inc. P.O. Box 279 Westford, MA 01886 (800) 828-1056	Full line of optical and nonoptical devices
Optical Designs, Inc. 14441 Memorial Drive, Suite 13 Houston, TX 77079 (713) 497-2988	Specialty line of Spitzberg magnifiers, behind-the-lens telescopes, and field enhancers
Precision Vision 745 North Harvard Avenue Villa Park, IL 60181 (630) 833-1454	Hyvärinen line of diagnostic charts and tests
Pulse Data International 6245 King Road Loomis, CA 95650 (916) 652-7253	Closed-circuit televisions, computer adaptations
Re-Kindle 5462 Memorial Drive, Suite 101 Stone Mountain, GA 30083 (800) 666-7484	Field-enhancement devices

See-More Vision Aiding Products P.O. Box 3413 Farmingdale, NY 11735 (800) 428-6673	Closed-circuit televisions
Spalding Magnifiers & Low Vision 7426 Tunbury Lane Houston, TX 77095 (888) 855-8666	Full line of optical and nonoptical devices Low vision instructional services
Telesensory Systems, Inc. 455 North Bernardo Avenue Mountain View, CA 94043-5237 (800) 804-8004	Closed-circuit televisions, large-print software
The Lighthouse, Inc. Lighthouse Low Vision Products 36-02 Northern Boulevard Long Island City, NY 11101 (800) 453-4923	Full line of optical and nonoptical devices Low vision instructional services
Unilens Corporation USA 10431 72nd Street North Largo, FL 33777 (800) 446-2020	Stick-on microscope bifocal
Visionics Corporation 1000 Boone Avenue North, Suite 600 Minneapolis, MN 55427 (800) 50-SIGHT	Low Vision Imaging System
Walters, Inc. 30423 Canwood Street, Suite 126 Agoura Hills, CA 91301 (818) 706-2902	Full line of optical devices
Xerox Adaptive Technologies 9 Centennial Drive Peabody, MA 01960 (508) 977-2000	Closed-circuit televisions

Appendix G:
Computer Access Resources

*Gregory L. Goodrich, Norine Krueger, Dan Nakamura,
Theresa Sacco, and Donalyn Warden*

This list is taken from *The Green Sheet: WBRC's Large-Print
Computer Access Resource List.*
Western Blind Rehabilitation Center
VA Palo Alto Health Care System
3801 Miranda Avenue
Palo Alto, CA 94304
(415) 493-5000
e-mail: goodrich@roses.stanford.edu

DOS AND WINDOWS-COMPATIBLE PRODUCTS

Product: Screen Magnifier/2   Price: $495
Company: IBM
Address: IBM Special Needs, 1000 NW 51st St.,
          Boca Raton, FL 33432
Telephone: (800) 426-7630
Compatibility: OS/2
System requirements: 386SX or higher
Video compatibility: VGA
Minimum RAM: 8 MB   Hard disk space: 1.2 MB
Magnification range: 2–32×
Comments: Compatible with OS/2, DOS,
          and Windows programs.

Product: Big for WordPerfect (DOS) 1.1   Price: $39
Company: Hexagon Products Presents
Address: P.O. Box 1295, Park Ridge, IL 60008-7295
Telephone: (708) 692-5555   e-mail: 76064-1776@compuserve.com
Compatibility: DOS
System requirements: 286 processor or better
Video compatibility: VGA

Minimum RAM: 1–4 MB (40 K memory resident)
Hard disk space: 100 K
Magnification range: 1.5–8.0×
Network compatible: No
Comments: Can be considered a utility in that it is a special-
purpose program only for WordPerfect. Similar
program available for Lotus 1-2-3.

Product: B-Edit   Price: $39
Company: Hexagon Products Presents
Address: P.O. Box 1295, Park Ridge, IL 60008-7295
Telephone: (708) 692-6555   e-mail: 76064-1776@compuserve.com
Compatibility: DOS
System requirements: 286 processor or better
Video compatibility: VGA
Minimum RAM: 1–4 MB (130 K memory resident)
Hard disk space: 250 K
Magnification range: 18-point type
Network compatible: No
Comments: Text editor, not word processor. Has most word-
processing commands with spellchecker, but not
really a document-formatting tool.

Product: B-Pop   Price: $35
Company: Hexagon Products Presents
Address: P.O. Box 1295, Park Ridge, IL 60008-7295
Telephone: (708) 692-5555   e-mail: 76064-1776@compuserve.com
Compatibility: DOS
System requirements: 286 processor or better
Video compatibility: VGA
Minimum RAM: 1–4 MB (30 K memory resident)
Hard disk space: 100 K
Magnification range: 1.5–8.0×
Network compatible: No
Comments: Memory-resident magnifying glass

Product: LPDOS   Price: $495
Company: Optelec
Address: P.O. Box 729, 6A Lyberty Way, Westford, MA 01886
Telephone: (800) 828-1056   Fax: (508) 692-6073
Compatibility: DOS
Speech compatible: Yes (JAWS, ASAP)
System requirements: 286 processor or better
Video compatibility: VGA
Minimum RAM: Not indicated   Hard disk space: 40K

Magnification range: 2–16×
Network compatible: Yes

Product: LPDOS Deluxe   Price: $595
Company: Optelec
Address: P.O. Box 729, 6A Lyberty Way, Westford, MA 01886
Telephone: (800) 828-1056   Fax: (508) 692-6073
Compatibility: DOS, Windows, Windows 95
Speech compatible: Yes (JAWS, ASAP)
System requirements: 286 processor or better
Video compatibility: VGA, SVGA
Minimum RAM: Not indicated   Hard disk space: 40K
Magnification range: 2–16× in Windows and DOS
Network compatible: Yes

Product: MAGic 1.33   Price: $295
Company: Microsystems Software, Inc. (Handiware Division)
Address: 600 Worcester Road, Framingham, MA 01701
Telephone: (800) 828-2600   Fax: (508) 879-1069
              e-mail: info@microsys.com
Compatibility: DOS, Windows, Windows 95
Speech compatible: Yes (IBM Screen Reader, JAWS)
System requirements: 386 processor or better
Video compatibility: VGA, SVGA
Minimum RAM: 4 MB recommended   Hard disk space: 500 K
Magnification range: 2–8× in Windows; 1.2–12.0× in DOS
Network compatible: Yes
Comments: Network-specific packages available. Site licenses, LAN-
              based network packages, and five- or 10-user laboratory
              packages are available for most products.

Product: MAGic 2.0   Price: $349
Company: Microsystems Software, Inc. (Handiware Division)
Address: 600 Worcester Road, Framingham, MA 01701
Telephone: (800) 828-2600   Fax: (508) 879-1069
              e-mail: info@microsys.com
Compatibility: DOS, Windows, Windows 95
Speech compatible: Yes (IBM Screen Reader, JAWS)
System requirements: 286 processor or better
Video compatibility: VGA, SVGA
Minimum RAM: 4 MB   Hard disk space: 230 K
Magnification range: 2–8× in Windows; 1.2–12.0× in DOS
Network compatible: Yes
Comments: Network-specific packages available

Product: Magnum GT   Price: $295
Company: Artic Technologies International Inc.
Address: 55 Park St, Troy, MI 48083
Telephone: (810) 588-7370   Fax: (810) 588-2650
Compatibility: DOS (up to 6.0), Windows 3.1
Speech compatible: Yes (WinVision and Business Vision)
System requirements: 286 processor or better
Video compatibility: EGA, VGA
Minimum RAM: 640 K   Hard disk space: 100 K
Magnification range: Up to 2× in Windows; up to 8× in DOS
Network compatible: Yes

Product: Magnum Deluxe   Price: $495
Company: Artic Technologies International Inc.
Address: 55 Park St, Troy, MI 48083
Telephone: (810) 588-7370   Fax: (810) 588-2650
Compatibility: DOS (up to 6.0); Windows 3.1
Speech compatible: Yes (WinVision and Business Vision)
System requirements: 286 processor or better
Video compatibility: EGA, VGA
Minimum RAM: 640 K   Hard disk space: 100 K
Magnification range: Up to 32× in Windows; up to 16× in DOS
Network compatible: Yes

Product: SuperVista (also called Vista SVGA)   Price: $2,495
Company: TeleSensory Systems Inc.
Address: 455 N. Bernardo Ave., Mountain View, CA 94039
Telephone: (800) 804-8004   Fax: (415) 335-1816
Compatibility: DOS, Windows
Speech compatible: Yes (DecTalk)
System requirements: 486 processor; vertical frequency
                     56–75 Hz refresh rate
Video compatibility: VGA, SVGA
Minimum RAM: 4 MB   Hard disk space: 15 K
Magnification range: 1.5–16.0×
Network compatible: Yes
Comments: Requires installation of TSI board

Product: VisAbility   Price: $495
Company: Ai Squared
Address: P.O. Box 669, Manchester Center, VT 05255
Telephone: (802) 362-3612   Fax: (802) 362-1670
Compatibility: DOS
Speech compatible: No
System requirements: 386 processor or better

Video compatibility: VGA
Minimum RAM: 4 MB (8 MB recommended)
Hard disk space: 2 MB
Comments: VisAbility allows the user to scan text into the computer for word processing and printing in large print from 1–8×. Scans both print and graphics.

Product: ZoomText   Price: $395
Company: Ai Squared
Address: P.O. Box 669, Manchester Center, VT 05255
Telephone: (802) 362-3612   Fax: (802) 362-1670
Compatibility: DOS
Speech compatible: No
System requirements: 386 processor or better
Video compatibility: VGA
Minimum RAM: 4 MB (8 MB recommended)
Hard disk space: 4 MB
Magnification range: 2–16× with smoothed characters
Network compatible: No

Product: ZoomText Plus   Price: $595
Company: Ai Squared
Address: P.O. Box 669, Manchester Center, VT 05255
Telephone: (802) 362-3612   Fax: (802) 362-1670
Compatibility: DOS, Windows
Speech compatible: No
System requirements: 386 processor or better
Video compatibility: VGA, SVGA
Minimum RAM: 4 MB (8 MB recommended)
Hard disk space: 4 MB
Magnification range: 2–16× with smoothed characters
Network compatible: No

MACINTOSH-COMPATIBLE PRODUCTS

Product: inLARGE 2.0a   Price: $195
Company: Berkeley Systems Inc.
Address: 2095 Rose St., Berkeley, CA 94709
Telephone: (510) 883-6280   Fax: (510) 883-6270
            e-mail: inlarge@berksys.com
Compatibility: Macintosh (except Power Macintosh models)
Speech compatible: Yes (outSPOKEN by Berkeley Systems)
System requirements: System 6.07 or higher
Video compatibility: Color or black-and-white monitors

Minimum RAM: 1 MB (more recommended)
Hard disk space: 350 K
Magnification range: 2–16×
Network compatible: Yes
Comments: Versions compatible with Power Macintosh computers are available. These are provided as free upgrades to owners of inLARGE 2.0a.

Index

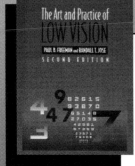
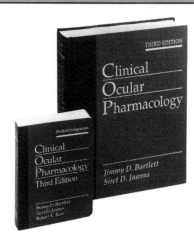